Workbook *for*

Egan's Fundamentals of Respiratory Care

Thirteenth Edition

Prepared by

Sandra T. Hinski, PhD, RRT
Dean, Career and Technical Education
Paradise Valley Community College
Phoenix, AZ

ELSEVIER

Elsevier
3251 Riverport Lane
St. Louis, Missouri 63043

WORKBOOK FOR EGAN'S FUNDAMENTALS OF RESPIRATORY CARE,   ISBN: 978-0-323-93200-4
THIRTEENTH EDITION

Copyright © 2025 by Elsevier Inc. All rights reserved.

No part of this publication may be reproduced or transmitted in any form or by any means, electronic or mechanical, including photocopying, recording, or any information storage and retrieval system, without permission in writing from the publisher, except that, until further notice, instructors requiring their students to purchase Workbook for Egan's Fundamentals of Respiratory Care by James K. Stoller, Albert J. Heuer, David L. Vines, Robert L. Chatburn, Sandra Hinski, and Eduardo Mireles-Cabodevila, may reproduce the contents or parts thereof for instructional purposes, provided each copy contains a proper copyright notice as follows: Copyright © 2025 by Elsevier Inc.

Details on how to seek permission, further information about the Publisher's permissions policies and our arrangements with organizations such as the Copyright Clearance Center and the Copyright Licensing Agency, can be found at our website: www.elsevier.com/permissions.

This book and the individual contributions contained in it are protected under copyright by the Publisher (other than as may be noted herein).

Notice

Practitioners and researchers must always rely on their own experience and knowledge in evaluating and using any information, methods, compounds or experiments described herein. Because of rapid advances in the medical sciences, in particular, independent verification of diagnoses and drug dosages should be made. To the fullest extent of the law, no responsibility is assumed by Elsevier, authors, editors or contributors for any injury and/or damage to persons or property as a matter of products liability, negligence or otherwise, or from any use or operation of any methods, products, instructions, or ideas contained in the material herein.

Previous editions copyrighted 2021, 2017, 2013, 2009, 2003, 1999.

Content Strategist: Melissa Rawe
Senior Content Development Specialist: Elizabeth McCormac
Publishing Services Manager: Deepthi Unni
Project Manager: Sheik Mohideen K

Printed in India

Last digit is the print number: 9   8   7   6   5   4   3   2   1

Working together
to grow libraries in
developing countries

www.elsevier.com • www.bookaid.org

For Charlie and Stella

Contents

Section I: Foundations of Respiratory Care, 1
Chapter 1: Early History of Respiratory Care, **1**
Chapter 2: The Profession of Respiratory Care, **4**
Chapter 3: Quality, Patient Safety, and Communication, **6**
Chapter 4: Principles of Infection Prevention and Control, **11**
Chapter 5: Ethical and Legal Implications of Practice, **17**
Chapter 6: Physical Principles of Respiratory Care, **22**
Chapter 7: E-Medicine in Respiratory Care, **28**
Chapter 8: Fundamentals of Respiratory Care Research, **30**

Section II: Applied Anatomy and Physiology, 33
Chapter 9: The Respiratory System, **33**
Chapter 10: The Cardiovascular System, **43**
Chapter 11: Ventilation, **47**
Chapter 12: Gas Exchange and Transport, **53**
Chapter 13: Solutions, Body Fluids, and Electrolytes, **61**
Chapter 14: Acid-Base Balance, **67**
Chapter 15: Regulation of Breathing, **75**

Section III: Assessment of Respiratory Disorders, 83
Chapter 16: Bedside Assessment of the Patient, **83**
Chapter 17: Interpreting Clinical and Laboratory Data, **92**
Chapter 18: Interpreting the Electrocardiogram, **97**
Chapter 19: Analysis and Monitoring of Gas Exchange, **105**
Chapter 20: Pulmonary Function Testing, **115**
Chapter 21: Review of Thoracic Imaging, **123**
Chapter 22: Flexible Bronchoscopy and the Respiratory Therapist, **132**
Chapter 23: Nutrition Assessment, **136**

Section IV: Review of Cardiopulmonary Disease, 143
Chapter 24: Pneumonia, **143**
Chapter 25: Obstructive Lung Disease: Chronic Obstructive Pulmonary Disease (COPD), Asthma, and Related Diseases, **149**
Chapter 26: Interstitial Lung Disease, **163**
Chapter 27: Pleural Diseases, **168**
Chapter 28: Pulmonary Vascular Disease, **177**
Chapter 29: Acute Respiratory Distress Syndrome (ARDS), **183**
Chapter 30: Respiratory Management of Trauma, Obesity, Near Drowning, and Burns, **188**
Chapter 31: Acute Heart Failure, **193**
Chapter 32: Lung Cancer, **196**
Chapter 33: Neuromuscular and Other Diseases of the Chest Wall, **203**
Chapter 34: Disorders of Sleep, **210**
Chapter 35: Neonatal and Pediatric Respiratory Disorders, **216**

Section V: Basic Therapeutics, 227
Chapter 36: Airway Pharmacology, **227**
Chapter 37: Airway Management, **238**
Chapter 38: Emergency Cardiovascular Life Support, **248**
Chapter 39: Humidity and Bland Aerosol Therapy, **257**
Chapter 40: Aerosol Drug Therapy, **265**
Chapter 41: Storage and Delivery of Medical Gases, **273**

Copyright © 2025, Elsevier, Inc. All rights reserved.

Chapter 42: Medical Gas Therapy, **281**
Chapter 43: Lung Expansion Therapy, **292**
Chapter 44: Airway Clearance Therapy (ACT), **298**

Section VI: Acute and Critical Care, 307
Chapter 45: Respiratory Failure and the Need for Ventilatory Support, **307**
Chapter 46: Mechanical Ventilators, **316**
Chapter 47: Physiology of Ventilatory Support, **321**
Chapter 48: Patient-Ventilator Interactions, **330**
Chapter 49: Initiating and Adjusting Invasive Ventilatory Support, **334**
Chapter 50: Noninvasive Ventilation, **344**
Chapter 51: Extracorporeal Life Support, **350**
Chapter 52: Monitoring the Patient in the Intensive Care Unit, **354**
Chapter 53: Discontinuing Ventilatory Support, **364**
Chapter 54: Neonatal and Pediatric Respiratory Care, **375**

Section VII: Patient Education and Long-Term Care, 385
Chapter 55: Patient Education and Health Promotion, **385**
Chapter 56: Cardiopulmonary Rehabilitation, **391**
Chapter 57: Respiratory Care in Alternative Settings, **399**
Chapter 58: Ethics and End of Life, **409**

Copyright © 2025, Elsevier, Inc. All rights reserved.

1 Early History of Respiratory Care

WORD WIZARD

Getting to know the terminology of respiratory care can be a challenge. Each chapter in this workbook starts with some word work to help you learn to "talk the talk" of a professional respiratory therapist and communicate with all members of the healthcare team.

Match the following terms to their definitions.

Definitions	Terms
_____ 1. Caregiver who acts as a physician extender after receiving additional education.	A. AARC
_____ 2. National professional association for respiratory care.	B. CoARC
_____ 3. Healthcare discipline that specializes in the promotion of optimum cardiopulmonary health.	C. NBRC
_____ 4. Name suggesting increased involvement in disease prevention and management and promotion of health and wellness.	D. cardiopulmonary system
_____ 5. One of the primary treatments for asthma uses this method of delivery.	E. respiratory care
_____ 6. Widely prescribed in hospitals by the 1940s and still a mainstay of respiratory care.	F. respiratory therapy
_____ 7. Organization responsible for the respiratory care credentialing examinations.	G. respiratory therapists
_____ 8. An iron lung is an example of this therapy that helps patients who cannot breathe.	H. oxygen therapy
_____ 9. Professional organization that accredits respiratory care schools and programs.	I. aerosol medications
_____ 10. Heart and lungs working together is the "bread and butter" of our profession.	J. mechanical ventilation
_____ 11. Method to test the ways that height, age, obesity, and disease alter lung function.	K. BOMA
_____ 12. Another name for the RT is this more formal term.	L. pulmonary function testing
_____ 13. Individual trained to deliver care to patients with heart and lung disease.	M. physician assistant
_____ 14. The AARC leadership receives formal input from this group on all matters and questions pertaining to patient care.	N. respiratory care practitioners

Copyright © 2025, Elsevier, Inc. All rights reserved.

Chapter 1 presented eight main objectives for learning. Test how well you understand these mysteries of history by providing short answers to these questions.

15. Define the respiratory care profession in your own words. How did the profession get started? Why are we here?

16. Describe how RT schools got started. What kinds of programs do they have now? How do these programs differ from those in the early days?

SUMMARY CHECKLIST

17. List the specialty sections of the AARC that provide recourses to members based on where they are employed and practice.

18. The AARC is the professional organization for the field. When was it originally started and what was it referred to then?

19. During the epidemics of the 1930s and 1950s, the iron lung was used extensively at a treatment for what disease?

Copyright © 2025, Elsevier, Inc. All rights reserved.

20. Describe at least four careers that would become possible for you as a result of baccalaureate or graduate education.

    A. _____

    B. _____

    C. _____

    D. _____

Copyright © 2025, Elsevier, Inc. All rights reserved.

2 The Profession of Respiratory Care

WORD WIZARD

The Key Terms in Chapter 2 are more complicated because they describe organizations, methods for disease management, and outcome monitoring.

Increase your understanding by matching the terms below to the Big Ideas.

Term	Big Idea
1. CoARC	_____ Responsible for quality of credentialing exams
2. The Joint Commission	_____ Responsible for quality of schools
3. Evidence-based medicine	_____ Uses meta-analyses to find best care
4. NBRC	_____ Uses site visits to check quality of care
5. ICRC	_____ Develops a worldwide code of ethics within respiratory care

MEET THE OBJECTIVES

Fill in your answers in the spaces provided.

6. Who is the primary leader of the respiratory therapy department?

7. How can protocols enhance the quality of respiratory care services?

8. What is the advance practice respiratory therapist?

4

Copyright © 2025, Elsevier, Inc. All rights reserved.

Complete the following statements by writing the correct information in the spaces provided.

9. What are the objectives of CoBGRTE?

10. What are protocols?

11. What is the highest credential in the respiratory care profession?

12. What organization is responsible for respiratory care credentialing examinations?

FOOD FOR THOUGHT

13. There has been a movement to move the entry to licensure to the RRT for all those seeking licensure for the first time. What does your state require for entry into practice?

5

Copyright © 2025, Elsevier, Inc. All rights reserved.

3 Quality, Patient Safety, and Communication

Fill in your answers in the spaces provided.

1. Briefly describe the four components of the PDSA cycle.

   A. _____

   B. _____

   C. _____

   D. _____

2. Briefly describe the five components of the DMAIC cycle.

   A. _____

   B. _____

   C. _____

   D. _____

   E. _____

3. Briefly describe the Hospital Value-Based Purchasing Program. How are the rewards for the program funded?

   _____

   _____

   _____

4. List the four components of a disease management program.

   A. _____

   B. _____

   C. _____

   D. _____

5. How can respiratory care plans be monitored for correctness?

Copyright © 2025, Elsevier, Inc. All rights reserved.

6. You are assisting in the ambulation of a patient receiving mechanical ventilation. What are the steps in moving the patient safely?

   A. _____

   B. _____

   C. _____

   D. _____

   E. _____

   F. _____

   G. _____

   H. _____

   I. _____

   J. _____

7. What are the three factors that determine the harmful effect of current?

   A. _____

   B. _____

   C. _____

8. Write the equation used to calculate current.

   _____

9. What physical effect should you suspect with 12 mA of current? Are there any factors that can change that effect?

   _____

   _____

10. As it relates to electrical devices, what is a ground?

    _____

11. What three conditions must exist for a fire to start?

    A. _____

    B. _____

    C. _____

12. What is the term used to describe a small current that enters the body through external catheters and may cause ventricular fibrillation?

Copyright © 2025, Elsevier, Inc. All rights reserved.

13. What does the acronym RACE stand for?

A. _____

B. _____

C. _____

D. _____

14. What is one thing the RT can do to help minimize fall risk for their patients?

_____

15. What do Gauss lines refer to?

_____

16. What does SBAR stand for?

A. _____

B. _____

C. _____

D. _____

17. Think about how you communicate during a patient hand-off. What could you do to improve the effectiveness of your message?

_____

18. How can you improve your listening skills?

_____

CASE STUDIES

Case 1

The physician orders ambulation for a patient who is receiving oxygen. The nurse asks you to assist. The patient is in bed wearing a nasal cannula running at 2 L/min.

19. What equipment will you need *before* you try to walk with this patient?

After 5 minutes of walking, you notice that the patient is breathing at a rate of 24 breaths/min and using his accessory muscles of ventilation. His skin appears sweaty, and he is exhaling through pursed lips.

20. What observations are important to note in this situation? What action would you take?

Copyright © 2025, Elsevier, Inc. All rights reserved.

Case 2

You are caring for a patient who is on a mechanical ventilator. You need to transport the patient to radiology for a CT scan. The nurse unplugs the IV pump and pulse oximeter from the *back* of each unit. The pumps and the pulse oximeter are now running on their battery systems. As you prepare to leave, you notice that the power cords are still plugged into the wall outlets. The physician and the nurse are anxious to get the transport under way.

21. Describe the actions you would take if you encountered this situation.

22. What potential conflict/communication problems exist? How would you deal with them?

WHAT DOES THE NBRC SAY?

Circle the best answer for the following multiple choice questions.

23. A respiratory therapist has completed SOAP charting in the progress notes following a bronchodilator treatment. While signing the chart form, she notices that the wrong amount for the medication has been entered. Which of the following actions should be done at this time?
    1. Draw one line through the error.
    2. Notify the physician of the error.
    3. Write "Error" and initial.
    4. Recopy the progress notes.
        A. 1 and 2
        B. 1 and 3
        C. 2 and 4
        D. 3 and 4

24. A patient with asthma has orders for albuterol by medication nebulizer every 2 hours. During the shift, the patient improves, and the order is changed to every 4 hours. In regard to the new frequency, what action should you take?
    1. Note the change in your charting.
    2. Inform the registered nurse of the order.
    3. Frequency will change during your shift.
        A. 1 and 2
        B. 1 and 3
        C. 2 and 3
        D. 1, 2, and 3

25. A patient's heart rate increases from 88 to 134 beats/min following a breathing treatment. After reassuring the patient, the respiratory therapist should
    A. discontinue the therapy.
    B. reduce the dosage of the medication.
    C. place the patient on oxygen.
    D. notify the physician.

Copyright © 2025, Elsevier, Inc. All rights reserved.

26. What do you think is the most common type of injury in health care?

27. On what shift do most injuries, accidents, and patient incidents occur?

Copyright © 2025, Elsevier, Inc. All rights reserved.

4 Principles of Infection Prevention and Control

Principles of Infection Prevention and Control

WORD WIZARD

Match the key definition with the correct term.

Definitions	Terms
_____ Infections that are acquired in the hospital.	A. Fomites
_____ Inanimate objects that help transfer pathogens.	B. Nosocomial
_____ Death of all microorganisms.	C. Sterilization
_____ Universal method of protection for health workers.	D. Disinfection
_____ Death of pathogenic microorganisms.	E. Standard precautions

MEET THE OBJECTIVES

Fill in your answers in the spaces provided.

1. What is a health care–associated infection?

   _____

2. A. What type of program is charged with reducing the risk of hospital-acquired infections (HAIs)?

   B. What do these program procedures involve?

      1. _____

      2. _____

      3. _____

3. List three elements that are required for infections to develop.

   A. _____

   B. _____

   C. _____

Copyright © 2025, Elsevier, Inc. All rights reserved.

4. A susceptible host may be elderly, have HIV, or be undergoing chemotherapy, but we can still reduce host susceptibility by focusing on employee health and chemoprophylaxis. List six vaccinations that might help you decrease the risk of transmitting an HAI.

A. _____

B. _____

C. _____

D. _____

E. _____

F. _____

5. Respiratory therapists must know the routes of disease transmission so we can avoid infection. What are the three **major** routes? Give an example of each.

	ROUTE	EXAMPLE
A.		
B.		
C.		

6. Define the following equipment processing definitions.

Term	Definition
Cleaning	
Disinfection, low-level	
Disinfection, intermediate-level	
Disinfection, high-level	
Sterilization	

7. List the three general barrier methods to prevent exposure to organisms. Describe a situation or identify an organism for which you (as a respiratory therapist) would need this type of protection.

A. _____

B. _____

C. _____

SUMMARY CHECKLIST

Complete the following statements by writing the correct information in the spaces provided.

8. What agent is an option for high-level disinfection of semicritical respiratory care equipment?

Copyright © 2025, Elsevier, Inc. All rights reserved.

9. Among respiratory care equipment, what type has the greatest potential to spread infection?

10. What fluid should be used for tracheal suctioning and filling nebulizers and humidifiers?

11. What protective equipment should be worn during any procedure that can generate splashes or sprays of body fluids?

12. What protective equipment is part of routine care when there is skin contact?

13. What is the maximum duration of time that an HME can safely be used?

Copyright © 2025, Elsevier, Inc. All rights reserved.   Chapter **4** **Principles of Infection Prevention and Control**

Case 1

You work in the surgical intensive care unit (ICU) of a large urban hospital. Over the past 2 days, a number of postoperative patients in the unit have developed serious *Staphylococcus aureus* infections.

14. Why do postoperative patients have an increased risk of infection?

15. What is the most common source of *S. aureus* organisms?_____

_____

16. Identify three ways to disrupt the route of transmission in this situation.

A. _____

B. _____

C. _____

Case 2

During the third day of your clinical rotation, you are assigned to a therapist who has an extremely heavy workload on a medical floor of the hospital. The therapist puts on gloves for each patient contact and asks you to do so also. When you go to wash your hands after the first treatment, the therapist tells you, "We don't have time for that, and besides the gloves will keep our hands clean."

17. Explain the role of gloves in protecting practitioners and preventing the spread of infection.

Case 3

A serious COVID-19 outbreak occurs in a crowded local prison facility. You are called to the emergency department as four of the sickest patients are being admitted together to your hospital for treatment.

18. By what route does COVID-19 spread?

Copyright © 2025, Elsevier, Inc. All rights reserved.

19. What conditions could have increased transmission of COVID-19 in this setting?

20. What kinds of precautions should be taken to prevent the spread of infection once these patients are admitted?

21. What is a challenging aspect of COVID-19 infection?

22. What should you do if enough private rooms with airborne precautions are not available for this group of patients?

WHAT DOES THE NBRC SAY?

Circle the best answer for the following multiple choice questions.

The following questions refer to this situation:
   A 72-year-old female patient with COPD has a tracheostomy tube in place following prolonged intubation and mechanical ventilation. She is currently in the medical intensive care unit. After you take her off the ventilator, you will need to set up a heated aerosol system with an F_iO_2 of 40%.

23. What type of water should be placed in the nebulizer?
   A. Distilled water
   B. Tap water
   C. Normal saline solution
   D. Sterile distilled water

Copyright © 2025, Elsevier, Inc. All rights reserved.

24. To help lower the risk of a nosocomial infection when using heated aerosol systems, the respiratory therapist should do which of the following?
    1. Label the equipment with the date and time it is started.
    2. Avoid draining the tubing to prevent contamination.
    3. Use aseptic technique during the initial setup.
    4. Use a filter or heat and moisture exchanger (HME) to reduce airborne bacteria.
    A. 1 and 3
    B. 1 and 2
    C. 2 and 4
    D. 3 and 4

25. The best way to prevent the spread of infection in the ICU is to
    A. ensure that sterilized equipment is used.
    B. wash your hands after every patient contact.
    C. wear gloves when you come in contact with body fluids.
    D. isolate infected patients.

FOOD FOR THOUGHT

26. One of your fellow students comes to clinical rotation with a cold. He asks you not to tell your clinical instructor because missed clinical days are hard to make up. What is your reaction to this situation? What are the potential problems with this scenario?

27. The college recommends that you get immunized against hepatitis B before attending clinical rotation. The consent form lists a number of possible side effects of the vaccine, and the vaccination is expensive. What are the pros and cons of vaccines? What will you choose?

Copyright © 2025, Elsevier, Inc. All rights reserved.

5 Ethical and Legal Implications of Practice

Complete the following paragraph by writing the correct terms in the spaces provided.

The two basic types of law in the United States are public law and civil law. Public law is further divided into administrative

law and _____ law. Health care facilities operate under a mountain of regulations set by government agen-

cies. Private, or _____, law protects citizens who feel they have been harmed. The individual who brings a

complaint is called the _____, and those accused of wrongdoing are known as _____. A(n)

_____ is a civil wrong. These cases could easily involve a health care practitioner. There are three types of

civil law cases. _____ is the failure to perform your duties competently. Cases in which the patient falls, is
given the wrong medication, or is harmed by equipment revolve around a provider's duty to anticipate harm and prevent
it from happening.

 Expert testimony, professional guidelines, or even circumstantial evidence can determine what a reasonable and pru-

dent respiratory therapist would have done in a given situation. The Latin term _____ ("the thing speaks
for itself") is sometimes invoked to show that harm occurred because of inappropriate care. When a professional fails to

act skillfully, breaches ethics, or performs below a reasonable standard, it is called _____. Wrongdoing

may be considered intentional or unintentional. Intentional acts include _____, or placing another person

in fear of bodily harm, and _____, or physical contact without consent. Other common intentional harm

occurs through _____, which is verbal defamation of character, and _____, which is written

defamation of character. Finally, information about patients is considered private, or _____, and cannot be
shared with anyone who is not involved in their care.

1. The basis of ethics is found in philosophy and is a science in itself. What is the fundamental question of ethics?

2. What is the one primary purpose of a professional code of ethics?

Copyright © 2025, Elsevier, Inc. All rights reserved.

3. Describe some of the information you might gather or consider before making a decision that involves ethics. For example, before discontinuing life support for a patient who is brain dead, what might you consider?

4. Health care is constantly changing and evolving in ways that affect ethical and legal decision making. Please discuss one example, such as managed care, and briefly explain how this new kind of medicine might shape our choices.

CASE STUDIES

Case 1

You get a chance to meet with your fellow students for lunch in the hospital cafeteria during a busy clinical day. One of your classmates is bursting with excitement as you sit down to eat. "You won't believe what I got to do today! I was taking care of Mr. Hunter, a patient in the intensive care unit (ICU), and he started to go bad, and we had to intubate. Then he coded, and I got to do CPR! It was so cool!"

5. What's the problem with this situation? What violation has your classmate committed?

6. What are the possible consequences of this scenario?

7. What action should you take?

Copyright © 2025, Elsevier, Inc. All rights reserved.

8. Is this situation simply a breach of ethics or a violation of law?

You receive an order to administer a bronchodilator to a 27-year-old asthma patient. The patient refuses the therapy, stating, "I just can't take any more of this today!" He appears alert and oriented.

9. Does the patient have a legal right to refuse in this case? Cite evidence from the text to justify your answer.

10. How would you respond to this situation?

11. What other action should you take at this time?

After finishing with the previous patient, you receive a stat call to the orthopedic floor. The registered nurse informs you they are having problems with a 76-year-old woman who recently had surgical repair of a broken hip. As you enter the room, you notice that she has removed her oxygen mask. She is breathing rapidly, and her color is not good. The pulse oximeter shows a saturation of 84%. When you try to get the patient to wear the oxygen mask, she screams at you to get out of the room.

12. Does the patient have a legal right to refuse in this case? Cite evidence from the text to justify your answer.

Copyright © 2025, Elsevier, Inc. All rights reserved.

13. How would you respond to this situation?

14. Would physical restraints be an option or a possible case of battery?

SUMMARY CHECKLIST

Complete the following statements by writing the correct information in the spaces provided.

15. What are the four dominant theories underlying modern ethics?

16. What type of law deals with the relationships of private parties and the government?

17. What type of law deals with the recognition and enforcement of the rights and duties of private individuals and organizations?

Copyright © 2025, Elsevier, Inc. All rights reserved.

18. What law protects citizens from civil liability for any errors they make while attempting to give emergency aid?

19. Where is the scope-of-practice statue identified?

FOOD FOR THOUGHT

20. What is the difference between an advance directive and a living will?

21. What is the False Claims Act (FCA)?

Copyright © 2025, Elsevier, Inc. All rights reserved. Chapter **5** **Ethical and Legal Implications of Practice**

6 Physical Principles of Respiratory Care

WORD WIZARD

Complete the following paragraph by writing the correct terms in the spaces provided.

Without humidity, our airways get irritated and mucus gets thick and difficult to expectorate. The actual amount, or weight, of water vapor in a gas is called _____ humidity. As respiratory therapists, we compare the weight of water vapor to the amount it could hold if the gas were fully saturated. This ratio of content to capacity is known as _____ humidity. You hear about this on the weather report every day. I'm more interested in how much vapor gas can hold inside the airways. This amount is called percent _____ humidity. When inspired gas has less than 100% of its capacity, a humidity _____ exists. Humidifiers are used to make up the difference. When you get a can of cold soda on a hot day, water droplets begin to form on the outside of the can. That's because the air around the can is cooling (cold air does not hold as much water vapor as warm air).

When air cools and gaseous water returns to a liquid form, we say that _____ has occurred. The opposite effect occurs when the drink warms. Water molecules escape from the liquid into the air. This process is called _____ and adds to the humidity in the air.

Heat moves in mysterious ways—four of them, to be precise. Newborn babies are especially sensitive to heat loss. Keeping a preemie warm can make the difference between life and death! When babies are born, we dry them off to prevent loss through _____.

Then they are wrapped in cloth to prevent _____, or loss that occurs from contact with a cooler object. Finally, we may put them in incubators. The incubator provides warmth in two ways. First, a special light _____ heat toward the baby. Second, warm air blows into the incubator. Transfer of heat through movement of fluids (or gas) is called _____.

MEET THE OBJECTIVES

1. Oxygen normally exists as a gas at sea level. What has to happen to turn gaseous oxygen into liquid oxygen for medical use?

2. What happens to the temperature when liquid oxygen is converted into gaseous oxygen?

Copyright © 2025, Elsevier, Inc. All rights reserved.

3. Describe the two major types of internal energy. Which form is most likely the cause of the internal energy of gases?

4. At sea level, what is the primary factor that determines the state of matter?

5. Liquid water can easily turn into its gaseous or vapor form. Water vapor content of gas is important for comfort and airway health. What factors affect the amount and rate of vaporization of water?

6. Explain why visible moisture, a mist, appears when you exhale on a cold day.

7. What is the name of the primary law that governs resistance, or opposition, to flow through the airway and the amount of pressure, or work, that must be performed to overcome resistance and move air in and out?

OBEY THE LAWS

This section provides some real examples of gas laws in action.

In the spaces provided, identify which law is being demonstrated.

Example 1
A registered pulmonary function technologist (RPFT) is performing lung testing on a patient. The patient inhales 1.5 L from the spirometer.

8. What will happen to the volume of gas inside the patient's lungs? _____

_____

9. What is the gas law? _____

Example 2
A home care respiratory therapist places an oxygen cylinder in a van so that she can take it to a client's house. The van catches on fire.

10. What will happen to the pressure inside the cylinder as it gets warmer? _____

_____

11. What is the gas law? _____

23

Copyright © 2025, Elsevier, Inc. All rights reserved.

Example 3

When you start to inhale, your diaphragm drops and your chest expands. In other words, you increase the size, or volume, of your chest.

12. What happens to the pressure inside your chest?

_____

13. What is the gas law? _____

TRY IT

Here are some safe, easy experiments you can perform in the laboratory at school or at home.

Experiment 1

Place a dry, empty *glass* soda bottle in the freezer for at least 15 minutes. Take the bottle out and *immediately* cover the mouth of the bottle with a balloon. Wait a few minutes and watch!

14. What happened to the balloon? _____

15. Which gas law is responsible for the result? _____

Experiment 2

Cut out a 1-inch-wide strip of notebook paper. Hold one end of the paper to your chin, just below your lip. Blow steadily across the top of the paper.

16. What happened to the paper? _____

17. What principle is responsible for this action? _____

Another experiment that shows this same principle can be accomplished with balloons. Blow up two round balloons and tie them off. Attach about 1 foot of string to each balloon. Tape the string to a stick (such as a ruler or yardstick) so the balloons are about 6 to 8 inches apart. Blow between the balloons.

18. What happened to the balloons? _____

Experiment 3

Get a coffee stirrer, an ordinary straw, and a big straw (like the kind you use for a milkshake). Now get two cups. Put some water in one cup. Put some honey in another. Suck the water up through each straw. Now try the honey. To make this more interesting, get a 6-foot length of oxygen-connecting tubing. Try the two fluids again!

19. Which tube is easiest to suck through? _____

20. Which fluid is easiest to suck up? _____

21. Which gas law explains all this? _____

Experiment 4

Surface tension can be a hard concept to grasp, but it is easy to demonstrate. Take a cup or glass and fill it with water up to the top. Slowly add more water until the cup is about to overflow. Observe the water surface as it sits slightly above the rim of the cup.

22. Which gas law explains your ability to fill a cup above the rim without its overflowing?

_____

Copyright © 2025, Elsevier, Inc. All rights reserved.

23. What is the name of the curved surface of the water?

_____

CASE STUDIES

Case 1

A respiratory therapist decides to attend the AARC International Congress. To get there, the therapist must travel by air. Before taking off, the flight attendant explains the oxygen system. The therapist pays attention when he sees the partial rebreathing mask. He also knows that something interesting happens to oxygenation at 30,000 feet.

24. What is the barometric pressure (P_B) and partial pressure of inspired oxygen (PiO_2) at this altitude?

P_B _____

PiO_2 _____

25. A properly fitting oxygen mask can deliver about 70% oxygen to passengers. What would the PiO_2 be while wearing the mask?

_____

26. Which gas law did you use to make these conclusions?

_____

Case 2

Respiratory therapists frequently draw arterial blood samples to measure the partial pressures of oxygen and carbon dioxide in the blood. Many patients have elevated or decreased body temperatures.

27. What effect does a fever have on these partial pressure readings?

_____

28. A normal arterial carbon dioxide pressure ($PaCO_2$) is 40 mm Hg (torr) at a body temperature of 37°C. Estimate the new $PaCO_2$ if the body temperature is 40°C.

29. Why is temperature correction of arterial blood gas readings controversial?

Copyright © 2025, Elsevier, Inc. All rights reserved.

30. Convert 30°C to degrees Kelvin.

    Formula _____

    Solution _____

    Answer _____

31. Convert 68°F to degrees Celsius.

    Formula _____

    Solution _____

    Answer _____

32. Convert 40°C to degrees Fahrenheit.

    Formula _____

    Solution _____

    Answer _____

33. At body temperature, gas has a saturated capacity of about 44 mg of water vapor per liter. If a gas has an absolute humidity of 22 mg/L, what is the relative humidity?

    Formula _____

    Solution _____

    Answer _____

34. What is the humidity deficit in Question 33?

    Formula _____

    Solution _____

    Answer _____

35. Convert a pressure reading of 10 millimeters of mercury (mm Hg) to centimeters of water (cm H_2O).

    Formula _____

    Solution _____

    Answer _____

36. Convert a pressure reading of 10 centimeters of water (cm H_2O) to kilopascals (kPa). Hint: It's okay to round off.

    Formula _____

    Solution _____

    Answer _____

37. Air is normally about 21% oxygen. Calculate the partial pressure of oxygen in air (PiO_2) when the barometric pressure is 760 mm Hg.

    Formula _____

    Solution _____

    Answer _____

Copyright © 2025, Elsevier, Inc. All rights reserved.

38. Now calculate the new PiO_2 that would result if the barometric pressure is 500 mm Hg.

Formula _____

Solution _____

Answer _____

SUMMARY CHECKLIST

39. Which temperature scale is used universally in health care around the world?

40. List the four ways heat can be transferred.

A. _____

B. _____

C. _____

D. _____

41. How is the total partial pressure of a mixture of gases determined?

WHAT DOES THE NBRC SAY?

42. A blood gas analyzer is being calibrated with a 5% mixture of carbon dioxide and balance nitrogen. If the barometric pressure is 747 mm Hg, what reading would be most correct for the CO_2 electrode of the analyzer?
    A. 35 mm Hg
    B. 37 mm Hg
    C. 7.47 mm Hg
    D. 74.7 mm Hg

43. What is the most significant factor affecting airway resistance?
    A. Airway length
    B. Airway radius
    C. Gas viscosity
    D. Gas flow rate

FOOD FOR THOUGHT

44. What property of liquid oxygen makes it especially difficult and potentially harmful to work with at home?

27

Copyright © 2025, Elsevier, Inc. All rights reserved.

7 E-Medicine in Respiratory Care

COMPUTERS IN HEALTH CARE

Clinicians use computers to help interpret data, reach a diagnosis, and automate certain aspects of patient care. Fill in your answers in the spaces provided.

1. What do EHR and EMR stand for? Define and explain the difference between the two.

   A. EHR: _____

   B. EMR: _____

   Define and explain: _____

   _____

   _____

2. What is a PACS and how does it help respiratory therapists in a critical care setting?

3. What is the CPOE system and how does it help respiratory therapists in a hospital setting?

   _____

   _____

   _____

4. What does the term "benchmarking" mean? How does a manager use benchmarking to assess performance?

5. Health care providers are using computers in the area of disease prevention. Tell us more about the following two applications of information technology. How will respiratory therapists use technology to better care for patients?

   A. Tobacco cessation: _____

   _____

   _____

   B. Disease management: _____

   _____

   _____

28

Copyright © 2025, Elsevier, Inc. All rights reserved.

6. What is telehealth?

7. What procedure commonly utilizes POCT?

8. Define health informatics.

9. What are KPIs used to indicate?

10. Define clinical decision support (CDS). Please list an example of CDS.

11. What is a root-cause analysis?

FOOD FOR THOUGHT

Smartphones and other handheld devices can be invaluable. There are many very useful medical applications for these devices, and many are free to download. For example, there is a program that allows users to look up almost any drug and check dosages, costs, side effects, and so on. Also available is a blood gas calculator, Henderson-Hasselbalch calculator, peak flow and PFT norms, cylinder duration—you name it. Many students buy handheld devices because there is no better digital tool. You can shoot video of procedures in the laboratory or take photos of equipment for study purposes. Plus, they fit in your pocket! (But remember, you should not take pictures in the hospital.)

Copyright © 2025, Elsevier, Inc. All rights reserved.

8 Fundamentals of Respiratory Care Research

WORD WIZARD

1. Fill in the definitions of the following key words.

	KEY WORD	DEFINITION
A.	Bibliographic database	
B.	PubMed	
C.	Portals	
D.	Synthesized database	
E.	Hypothesis	
F.	Research protocols	

HOW TO BE A RESEARCHER

2. List, in correct order, the outline a research paper typically follows.

A. _____

B. _____

C. _____

D. _____

E. _____

3. Which section of a research paper explains what was done to answer the research question?

_____

4. What does IRB stand for? What is its purpose? _____

5. What are *peer reviewers* and what is their purpose regarding research papers?

_____

_____

6. What three outcome recommendations can a peer reviewers give to the journal editor about the submitted research paper?

A. _____

B. _____

C. _____

Copyright © 2025, Elsevier, Inc. All rights reserved.

7. Try to develop a study idea. Choose and define a research topic area and write it down. _____

_____

8. Go to the library website of your educational institution and use a bibliographic database to research your idea. Attempt the following activity.

   A. Go to the following website: https://pubmed.ncbi.nlm.nih.gov

   B. Enter one word in the first search field and click "Search." (Make sure the box to the left of the search field has PubMed displayed.) How many results did you get? _____

   C. Using the tab on the left column, limit your results to those published since 2022. How many results did you get? _____

   D. What is one way you can narrow your search? _____

   E. Now, add an additional key word to your initial key word in the search field using the word "AND" to separate the words. How many results did you get? (Hint: Look up what a Boolean operator is.) _____

   F. Under the search field click on the "Advanced" link. What happens? _____

   G. Find an article, open it, and evaluate the sources using the following categories.
      i. Relevance
        1. Does the information relate to your topic or question?
        2. What is the intended audience?
      ii. Currency
        1. When was the article published?
      iii. Authority (Remember, scholarly articles are written by experts and reviewed by experts!)
        1. What are the author's credentials or organizational affiliations?
        2. Is the research sponsored by a particular organization/company/agency?
      iv. Accuracy
        1. Is the information supported by evidence?
        2. Are there any spelling or grammatical errors?
      v. Purpose
        1. What is the purpose of the information? To inform? Teach? Sell a product? Persuade?
        2. Are there any political, ideological, institutional, or personal biases?
        3. Does the point of view appear to be objective and impartial?

   H. Does your educational institution have any expert tools to aid in creating citations? What is a common citation format for peer-reviewed articles? (Hint: Make an appointment with a librarian for help. They are a great resource!)

Copyright © 2025, Elsevier, Inc. All rights reserved.

Chapter **8** **Fundamentals of Respiratory Care Research**

9 | The Respiratory System

WORD WIZARD

Fill in the box below regarding medical terminology.

	MEDICAL TERMINOLOGY	IN PLAIN LANGUAGE, PLEASE
A.		Tiny air sacs for gas exchange
B.		Place where trachea splits into R+L
C.	Cilia	
D.		Primary muscle of breathing
E.	Epiglottis	
F.		Hole that opens into your windpipe
G.	Hilum	
H.		Voice box
I.	Pharynx	
J.		Wrapping that lines the lungs
K.	Sternum	
L.		Windpipe

FETAL FACTS

1. During what stage and week of development is alveolar capillary surface area considered sufficient to support extrauterine life?

   Stage: _____

   Week: _____

2. What is the primary organ of gas exchange for the fetus? _____

   _____

33

Copyright © 2025, Elsevier, Inc. All rights reserved.

3. Describe the umbilical cord blood vessels.

4. The fetus lives in a relatively hypoxic environment. What is considered to be a major factor that enables the fetus to survive under these conditions? _____

5. About half of the blood entering the right atrium is shunted to the left atrium via what structure?

   _____

6. Explain why fetal pulmonary vascular resistance is so high.

7. What percentage of blood entering the pulmonary artery actually flows through the lungs? Where does the rest of the blood go?

   _____

8. Describe the events that occur in the first few breaths after birth in terms of transpulmonary pressure, blood gases, and circulatory changes.

9. Compare the development of lung structures in newborns and adults.

   A. Number of alveoli

   B. Surface area of the lung

Copyright © 2025, Elsevier, Inc. All rights reserved.

10. Compare the head and upper airway of adults and infants.

	ANATOMY	INFANTS	ADULT
A.	Head		
B.	Tongue		
C.	Nasal passages		
D.	Larynx		
E.	Narrow point		
F.	Dead space		
G.	Airways		

11. Most infants breathe exclusively through what part of the airway? _____

12. Explain why infant lung volumes are relatively lower than those of adults.

13. What does it mean when an infant is grunting?

14. Why do infants experience severe hypoxemia more readily than adults?

Copyright © 2025, Elsevier, Inc. All rights reserved.

Identify the structures labeled in these figures.

15. What's in a chest? Label the bones in this anterior view of the thorax.

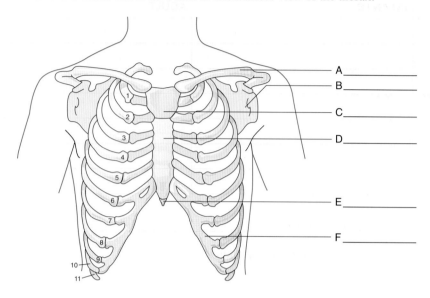

A_____

B_____

C_____

D_____

E_____

F_____

16. Label the imaginary lines on the anterior chest wall.

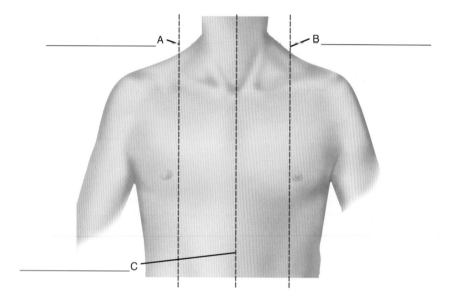

_____ A

B_____

_____ C

Copyright © 2025, Elsevier, Inc. All rights reserved.

17. Label the imaginary lines on the lateral chest wall.

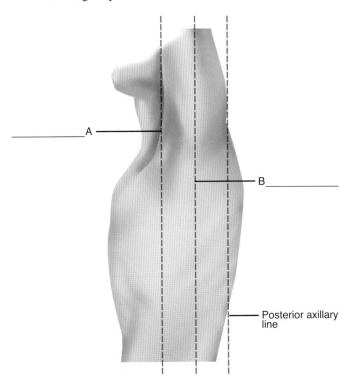

_____ A

B_____

Posterior axillary line

18. Identify and label the muscles of ventilation.

A _____
_____
_____

B _____

D_____

Internal intercostal

C _____

Sternum

E _____

F _____

Transverse abdominus

G _____

Internal obliques

Copyright © 2025, Elsevier, Inc. All rights reserved.

19. Label the structures of the upper airway and oral cavity.

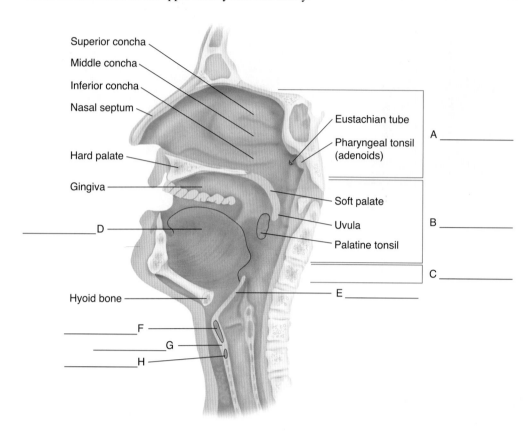

Superior concha

Middle concha

Inferior concha

Nasal septum

Hard palate

Gingiva

D _____

Hyoid bone

F _____

G

H

Eustachian tube

Pharyngeal tonsil (adenoids)

A _____

Soft palate

Uvula

B _____

Palatine tonsil

C _____

E _____

20. Label the anterior view of the larynx.

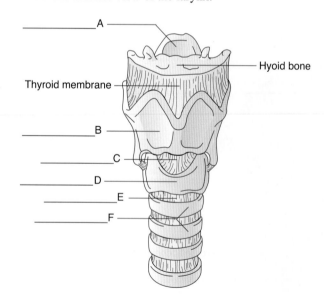

A _____

Hyoid bone

Thyroid membrane

B _____

C _____

D _____

E _____

F _____

Copyright © 2025, Elsevier, Inc. All rights reserved.

21. Label the respiratory cilia.

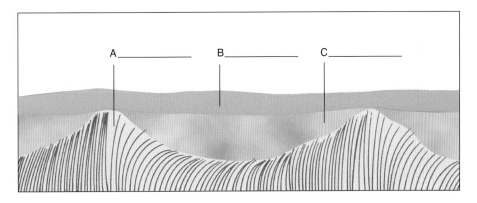

A_____ B_____ C_____

22. Label the cross-sectional sketch of the cells and organization of the alveolar septa.

Connective tissue entrance ring

Interstitial space

D_____

Endothelial cell } Capillary

A_____

B_____

E_____

F_____

C_____

Connective tissue fibers

Interstitial cell

Copyright © 2025, Elsevier, Inc. All rights reserved.

23. *Fill in the following chart as it relates to the descriptions of various anatomic structures*

Anterior, anteriorly, ventral	
Posterior, posteriorly, dorsal	
Anteroposterior	
Lateral, laterally	
Medial, medially	

MEET THE OBJECTIVES

Fill in your answers in the spaces provided.

24. List the nerves that innervate the diaphragm, intercostal muscles, and larynx. State the origin of these nerves and describe what will happen if they are damaged.

25. Describe the pathway gas follows as it is conducted through the lower airway.

SUMMARY CHECKLIST

26. What is the primary muscle of ventilation?

27. What does the upper respiratory tract do?

28. Is normal exhalation active or passive?

29. Describe what happens during forced exhalation.

Copyright © 2025, Elsevier, Inc. All rights reserved.

30. List a function of the diaphragm other than ventilation.

CASE STUDIES

Case 1

A respiratory instructor is lecturing on anatomy of the lung when, completely by coincidence, she slips, and a sharp pencil punctures her right chest. The students gather around their fallen facilitator to discuss the anatomic consequences of this tragedy.

31. What could happen to the lung on the affected side?

32. What could happen to the pleural space on the affected side?

33. What is this condition called? _____

34. What is the treatment for this condition?

_____

Case 2

A registered respiratory therapist (RRT) is working the night shift at a large urban medical center. As he makes his rounds, he hears loud snoring coming from a patient's room. Even though snoring is a commonly heard sound at night, the RRT stops to investigate.

35. What anatomic change results in snoring?

36. What is OSA, and how is it treated?

Copyright © 2025, Elsevier, Inc. All rights reserved.

37. What is the similarity between snorers and unconscious victims who require resuscitation?

38. How would you approach management of the airway of an unconscious person?

FOOD FOR THOUGHT

What happens to these structures when disease is present?

39. What happens to the airways and alveoli when a patient is having an acute episode of asthma?

40. What changes to the airways and alveoli occur in emphysema?

Copyright © 2025, Elsevier, Inc. All rights reserved.

10 The Cardiovascular System

Match the following terms to their definitions as they apply to respiratory care.

Terms	Definitions
_____ 1. Afterload	A. Membranous sac that surrounds the heart
_____ 2. Automaticity	B. Stroke volume multiplied by heart rate
_____ 3. Baroreceptors	C. Ventricular stretch provided by end-diastolic volume
_____ 4. Cardiac output	D. Biologic sensors that monitor arterial blood pressure
_____ 5. Chemoreceptors	E. Pathologic narrowing or constriction
_____ 6. Pericardium	F. Force against which the ventricle pumps
_____ 7. Preload	G. Biologic sensors that monitor arterial blood oxygen
_____ 8. Stenosis	H. Ability to initiate a spontaneous electrical impulse

MEET THE OBJECTIVES

9. Where is the mitral valve located? What effect can mitral valve stenosis have on the lungs?

10. Explain how specialized heart muscle tissue allows the muscle cells in the ventricle to contract in a coordinated and efficient manner.

11. Compare and contrast local control of blood vessels with central control mechanisms.

43

Copyright © 2025, Elsevier, Inc. All rights reserved.

12. Describe how the cardiovascular system responds to exercise and blood loss by balancing blood volume and vascular resistance.

13. Match the mechanical events to their corresponding electrical events in the normal cardiac cycle.

	ELECTRICAL EVENT	CARDIAC EVENT (MECHANICAL)
A.	P wave	
B.	QRS	
C.	T wave	

SUMMARY CHECKLIST

Complete the following questions by writing the correct information in the spaces provided.

14. The _____ system consists of the heart and vascular network, which maintain _____ by regulating the distribution of blood flow in the body.

15. What factors influence cardiac output?

16. Under conditions of increased demand, how is stable flow maintained?

17. What does the heart and vascular systems ensure?

18. How is blood pressure is regulated?

19. What effect will an increase in heart rate likely produce?

Copyright © 2025, Elsevier, Inc. All rights reserved.

CASE STUDIES

Case 1

A 57-year-old patient is admitted to the coronary care unit with a diagnosis of mitral stenosis. The patient is breathing rapidly and complains of shortness of breath. Her pulse oximetry readings reveal hypoxemia. Auscultation reveals inspiratory crackles in the posterior lower lobes.

20. Describe mitral valve stenosis. _____

21. What mechanical events are occurring to cause pulmonary edema and stiffening of the lung tissue?

22. What action should the respiratory therapist take at this time? _____

_____

Case 2

A respiratory care student is giving an aerosolized bronchodilator to a 27-year-old patient with asthma. Breath sounds reveal bilateral expiratory wheezing. The pulse oximeter shows 98% saturation on room air. The student notices the heart rate rising from 82 to 98 beats/min during the therapy.

23. What are the effects of sympathetic and parasympathetic stimulation on the sinus node in the heart?

    A. _____

    B. _____

24. Describe the two ways that medications can produce bronchodilation.

    A. _____

    B. _____

25. Based on this information, why would you expect increased heart rate to be a common side effect of some medications that cause bronchodilation?

WHAT DOES THE NBRC SAY?

Circle the best answer for the following questions.

26. A patient has a heart rate of 70 beats/min and a stroke volume of 60 ml with each contraction of the ventricle. What is the approximate cardiac output in liters per minute?
    A. 3.6 L/min
    B. 4.2 L/min
    C. 5.0 L/min
    D. 6.0 L/min

45

27. Calculate systemic vascular resistance if mean arterial pressure is 90 mm Hg, central venous pressure (CVP) is 10 mm Hg, and cardiac output is 4 L/min.
    A. 2.5 mm Hg/L/min
    B. 8.6 mm Hg/L/min
    C. 20 mm Hg/L/min
    D. 22.5 mm Hg/L/min

28. What is the ejection fraction if stroke volume is 50 ml and end-diastolic volume is 75 ml?
    A. 50%
    B. 66%
    C. 75%
    D. 150%

FOOD FOR THOUGHT

29. What four mechanisms combine to promote venous return to the heart?

    A. _____

    B. _____

    C. _____

    D. _____

30. What is meant by the "thoracic pump"? What effect can positive pressure ventilation have on venous return to the chest?

Copyright © 2025, Elsevier, Inc. All rights reserved.

11 Ventilation

Label the following diagram to help improve your understanding of these pressure changes.

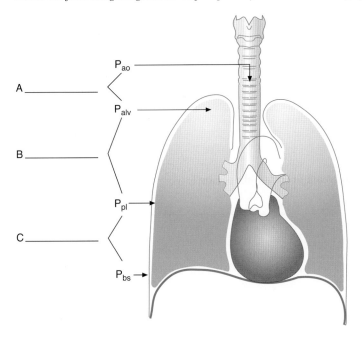

Pressures, volumes, and flows involved in ventilation. (Modified from Martin L: *Pulmonary physiology in clinical practice: the essentials for patient care and evaluation*, St. Louis, 1987, Mosby.)

1. Write out the definition of each gradient.

   A. Transrespiratory Pressure: _____

   B. Transpulmonary Pressure: _____

   C. Transthoracic Pressure: _____

47

Copyright © 2025, Elsevier, Inc. All rights reserved.

Questions

2. Fill in the missing pressures for the apex and base of the lung.

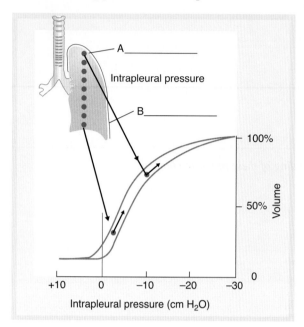

3. Where does the bulk of ventilation go during a normal breath in an upright person?

_____

Copyright © 2025, Elsevier, Inc. All rights reserved.

4. List the four factors that contribute to the work of breathing.

A. _____

B. _____

C. _____

D. _____

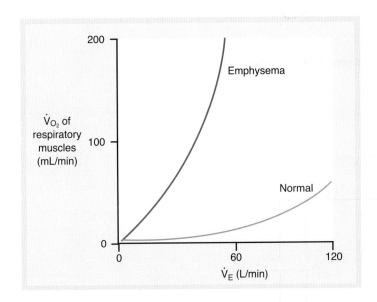

5. Why is the compliance of the lung tissue itself increased in emphysema?

6. What important change occurs in the airway of patients with COPD and asthma to increase the resistance? Which airways are usually involved?

7. What class of medications can respiratory therapists use to reduce airway resistance in asthma?

_____

8. What does it mean when you see active exhalation in your patient?

Copyright © 2025, Elsevier, Inc. All rights reserved.

9. What happens to persons with spinal cord injuries who cannot use their abdominal muscles?

10. Describe what happens to alveolar ventilation in healthy individuals when they increase respiratory rate or decrease tidal volume.

11. What is the optimal pattern of breathing for patients with obstructive airway diseases?

12. Label the types of dead space in this diagram.

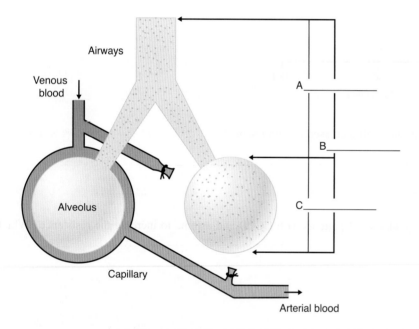

13. A. What is the normal percentage of anatomic dead space for each breath?
    B. What is the value used to calculate average anatomic dead space?

14. What type of ventilatory pattern will be seen with significantly increased dead space?

Copyright © 2025, Elsevier, Inc. All rights reserved.

15. What is the difference between *hyperventilation* and *hyperpnea*?

16. Calculate exhaled minute ventilation for a patient who has a tidal volume of 800 ml and a frequency of 8 breaths/min.

    Formula _____

    Calculation _____

    Answer _____

17. Calculate anatomic dead space for a patient who is 6 feet tall and weighs 180 lb.

    Formula _____

    Calculation _____

    Answer _____

18. Calculate alveolar minute ventilation using the data from Problems 16 and 17.

    Formula _____

    Calculation _____

    Answer _____

19. Calculate the physiologic dead space using the Bohr equation if $PaCO_2$ is 60 mm Hg and $PECO_2$ is 30 mm Hg.

    Formula _____

    Calculation _____

    Answer _____

WHAT DOES THE NBRC SAY?

Circle the best answer for the following multiple-choice questions.

20. The minute volume for a 68-kg (150-lb) patient who has a respiratory rate of 12 breaths/min and a tidal volume of 600 ml would be
    A. 4.8 L.
    B. 5.4 L.
    C. 6.0 L.
    D. 7.2 L.

21. The estimated alveolar minute ventilation for an 82-kg (180-lb) patient who has a respiratory rate of 10 breaths/min and a tidal volume of 500 ml would be
    A. 3.2 L.
    B. 3.5 L.
    C. 4.8 L.
    D. 5.0 L.

Copyright © 2025, Elsevier, Inc. All rights reserved.

22. Which of the following statements describes a lung unit with a long time constant?
    A. They take longer to fill and to empty than units with normal compliance and resistance.
    B. They fill and empty more rapidly than lung units with normal compliance and resistance.
    C. They take longer to fill and empty more rapidly than lung units with normal compliance and resistance.
    D. Time constants have no bearing on the filling or emptying of lung units.

23. Determine the physiologic dead space percentage for a patient with an arterial CO_2 of 40 mm Hg and an exhaled CO_2 of 30 mm Hg.
    A. 0.25
    B. 0.33
    C. 0.50
    D. 0.75

Copyright © 2025, Elsevier, Inc. All rights reserved.

12 Gas Exchange and Transport

MATHEMATICS

1. Calculate alveolar oxygen tension for Patient A breathing room air with a barometric pressure of 760 mm Hg. F_iO_2 is 21% and $PaCO_2$ is 40 mm Hg.

   Formula _____

   Solution _____

   Answer _____

2. If Patient A has an arterial PO_2 of 90 mm Hg, what is the A–a gradient?

   Formula _____

   Solution _____

   Answer _____

3. Calculate alveolar O_2 tension for Patient B breathing 60% O_2 (P_B = 760 mm Hg, CO_2 = 40 mm Hg).

   Formula _____

   Solution _____

   Answer _____

4. If Patient B has an arterial PO_2 of 90 mm Hg, what is the A–a gradient?

   Formula _____

   Solution _____

   Answer _____

5. Explain the difference in respiratory status between Patient A and Patient B based on the previous data.

Copyright © 2025, Elsevier, Inc. All rights reserved.

6. List the three barriers to diffusion.

   A. _____

   B. _____

   C. _____

7. What is the main force driving a gas across the alveolar-capillary membrane?

8. Calculate O_2 content for Patient 1 with an Hb of 15 g/dL, SaO_2 of 97%, and PaO_2 of 100 mm Hg.

   Formula _____

   Solution _____

   Answer _____

9. Calculate O_2 content for Patient 2 with an Hb of 15 g, SaO_2 of 80%, and PaO_2 of 50 mm Hg.

   Formula _____

   Solution _____

   Answer _____

10. Calculate O_2 content for Patient 3 with an Hb of 10 g, SaO_2 of 97%, and PaO_2 of 100 mm Hg.

   Formula _____

   Solution _____

   Answer _____

Fill in the correct values for partial pressure of O_2 and saturation (with a normal pH) on the chart below.

	PaO_2	SaO_2
11.	40 mm Hg	
12.		80%
13.	60 mm Hg	
14.		97%

Copyright © 2025, Elsevier, Inc. All rights reserved.

Fill in the correct answers for how the curve will shift in the following chart:

	Factor	Shift
15.	Acidosis	
16.	Hypothermia	
17.	High 2,3-diphosphoglycerate (2,3-DPG)	
18.	Fever	
19.	Hypercapnia	
20.	Carboxyhemoglobin	

GAS EXCHANGE

The following questions will test your knowledge of the causes of poor gas exchange.

21. What term is used to describe the inadequate delivery of O_2 to the tissues?

22. What term is used to describe a low level of O_2 in the blood?

23. What is the term used to describe what occurs when blood passes through areas of the lung that have no ventilation?

24. What type of imbalances is the most common cause of low blood O_2 in patients with lung disease?

25. What type of defect do patients with pulmonary fibrosis have that results in low blood O_2 levels?

26. What must be present for gas exchange to occur between the alveoli and pulmonary capillaries?

Copyright © 2025, Elsevier, Inc. All rights reserved.

27. What is the term used to describe a localized reduction in blood flow to tissues that can result in tissue death?

28. What effect could an increased dead space ventilation have on the levels of CO_2 in the blood?

29. What is a possible cause for inadequate minute or alveolar ventilation in a drug overdose?

30. Does oxygen or carbon dioxide have a greater alveolar membrane permeability?

WHAT DOES THE NBRC SAY?

Circle the best answer for each of the following multiple-choice questions.

31. A blood gas measurement in a patient reported to be breathing room air reveals the following results:

pH	7.45
$PaCO_2$	30 mm Hg
PaO_2	150 mm Hg

In regard to these data, the respiratory therapist should
A. report the results to the physician.
B. redraw the sample because of air contamination.
C. check if the patient is on O_2.
D. place the patient on O_2.

32. Calculate O_2 content for a patient with the following data:

Hb	10 g
PaO_2	80 mm Hg
SaO_2	95%

A. 12.73 ml O_2/dL
B. 12.97 ml O_2/dL
C. 13.40 ml O_2/dL
D. 13.64 ml O_2/dL

33. Calculate PAO_2 for a patient with the following data:

P_B	747 mm Hg
F_iO_2	0.21
PaO_2	95 mm Hg
$PaCO_2$	40 mm Hg
SaO_2	97%

A. 97 mm Hg
B. 103 mm Hg
C. 107 mm Hg
D. 117 mm Hg

Copyright © 2025, Elsevier, Inc. All rights reserved.

34. A man is brought to the emergency department from a house fire. He is conscious and in obvious distress on 6 L of O_2 via nasal cannula. His heart rate is 136 beats/min, respiration is 26 breaths/min, and blood pressure is 160/100 mm Hg. The pulse oximeter reading is SpO_2 100%. He has no cyanosis but complains of dyspnea. What abnormality of hemoglobin is most likely to be the source of the clinical problem?
   A. HbCO
   B. HbS
   C. Anemia
   D. HbF

CASE STUDIES

Case 1

A 29-year-old housewife is brought to the emergency department following exposure to smoke during a house fire. She is breathing at a rate of 30 breaths/min. Her heart rate is 110 beats/min. Blood pressure is 160/110 mm Hg. The patient complains of headache and nausea. The pulse oximeter reading shows a saturation of 100%.

35. Why are pulse oximeter readings unreliable in this setting? _____

_____

36. What is wrong with this patient?

37. What action would you take at this time?

Case 2

A patient is brought back to the unit following major surgery after a motorcycle accident. He was given a massive blood transfusion to replace loss from both the trauma and the surgical procedure. The pulse oximeter reading is 96% on room air, but the nurse has requested your evaluation because of the patient's clinical condition. You find him sitting up and breathing 32 times per minute. He has tachycardia and tachypnea and complains of difficulty breathing. Breath sounds are clear on auscultation.

38. The patient's clinical signs are consistent with what gas exchange abnormality?

_____

39. What is one of the potential problems with banked blood?

_____

40. Name some of the other possible causes of the patient's distress.

Copyright © 2025, Elsevier, Inc. All rights reserved.

Chapter **12** **Gas Exchange and Transport**

41. What diagnostic procedure could you recommend? _____

_____

A woman is admitted with a diagnosis of pneumonia. Arterial blood gas measurements reveal a pH of 7.55, $PaCO_2$ of 25 mm Hg, PaO_2 of 75 mm Hg, and SaO_2 of 94%. She complains of feeling short of breath. Laboratory data reveal a hemoglobin level of 8 g/dL.

42. Interpret these blood gas findings in terms of gas exchange.

43. What other laboratory information plays a key role in helping to determine O_2 content?

_____

44. What is absolute anemia, and how is it treated?

A young man has been brought to the emergency department by paramedics after an accidental overdose of narcotics at a party. The patient is unconscious and has a respiratory rate of 8 breaths/ min. The pulse oximeter shows a saturation of 85%.

45. Why would CO_2 be elevated in this patient?

46. Why is the patient's O_2 saturation so low?

Copyright © 2025, Elsevier, Inc. All rights reserved.

47. What does the movement of gas between the lungs and the tissues depend on?

48. How does alveolar ventilation and PCO_2 vary?

49. Why does lactic acid form when tissues are hypoxic?

50. Blood carries a small amount of dissolved O_2 in the plasma. Where is most of O_2 carried?

51. List five causes of a decreased PaO_2, or O_2, level in arterial blood.

    A. _____

    B. _____

    C. _____

    D. _____

    E. _____

52. How is most of CO_2 in your blood is transported?

53. What may be the result of a decrease in either arterial blood O_2 content or flow?

54. What happens when the minute ventilation is decreased or when dead space ventilation is increased?

59

Copyright © 2025, Elsevier, Inc. All rights reserved.

55. What is the classic example of dysoxia? _____

_____

56. When does tissue O_2 consumption become dependent on O_2 delivery? _____

_____

Copyright © 2025, Elsevier, Inc. All rights reserved.

13 Solutions, Body Fluids, and Electrolytes

Write your answer in the spaces provided.

Definitions		Terms
1. _____ A compound that gives off H^+ in water.		A. Acid
2. _____ The opposite of inactive transport; movement across membranes.		B. Active transport
3. _____ Negatively charged ion; Cl^- and HCO_3^- are common in the body.		C. Normal solution
4. _____ A compound that gives off OH^- in water.		D. Solvent
5. _____ Minimizing the change in pH.		E. Solute
6. _____ Positively charged ion; Na^+ and K^+ are common in the body.		F. Base
7. _____ A substance with big molecules that hold water and also an evenly dispersed mixture or gel.		G. Cations
8. _____ Something you use to water down a medication or solution.		H. Hypertonic
9. _____ The medium you dissolve something into.		I. Isotonic
10. _____ The stuff that gets dissolved.		J. Solution
11. _____ A stable mixture of two substances. Heat helps make this happen.		K. Diluent
12. _____ A really weak solution.		L. Colloid
13. _____ A solution holding as much as it can.		M. Dilute solution
14. _____ The standard solution with 1 mEq/L.		N. Hypotonic
15. _____ Has the same amount of salt as your body fluids.		O. Buffering
16. _____ Saltier than your body fluids.		P. Saturated solution
17. _____ Low salt or no salt.		Q. Anions

WATER, WATER EVERYWHERE

18. Rank the relative amount of water in the following individuals. Put "1" by the group with the lowest percentage of body water and "5" by the group with the largest percentage of body water.

_____ Males

_____ Newborns

_____ Children

_____ Females

_____ Obese individuals

Copyright © 2025, Elsevier, Inc. All rights reserved.

19. List subdivisions and give the relative amount (%) of water in each area.

COMPARTMENT	% H₂O
A. Intracellular	
B. Extracellular	
1.	
2.	
3.	

20. List the predominantly extracellular electrolytes.

   A. _____

   B. _____

   C. _____

21. List the predominantly intracellular electrolytes.

   A. _____

   B. _____

   C. _____

   D. _____

22. What amount of water can be lost through fever?

23. Lost water is regained by two main methods. List these sources of liquids and give amounts.

	SOURCE	AMOUNT/DAY
A. Ingestion		
1.		
2.		
B. Metabolism		

ACID-BASE BASICS

24. If a patient ingested bicarbonate for stomach problems and the pH went up from 7.0 to 8.0, how much more alkaline did the body become?

Copyright © 2025, Elsevier, Inc. All rights reserved.

25. What equation is used to calculate pH? Write it out to help remember it.

    A. Name

    B. Equation

ELECTRIFYING INFORMATION

26. List the seven major electrolytes and their primary purposes in the body.

	ELECTROLYTE	SYMBOL	PURPOSE
A.			
B.			
C.			
D.			
E.			
F.			
G.			

Match the value to the chemical in the list below.

27. _____ bicarbonate   A. 140 mEq/L

28. _____ calcium   B. 24 mEq/L

29. _____ chloride   C. 4.0 mEq/L

30. _____ magnesium   D. 5.0 mEq/L

31. _____ phosphorus   E. 100 mEq/L

32. _____ potassium   F. 2.0 mEq/L

33. _____ sodium   G. 1.4 mEq/L

63

Copyright © 2025, Elsevier, Inc. All rights reserved.

Complete the chart below to match up disorders, causes, and symptoms of electrolyte disturbances.

	IMBALANCE	CAUSE	SYMPTOM
34.		Sweating	
35.	Hypokalemia		
36.		Starvation	Diaphragmatic weakness
37.	Hypercalcemia		
38.		Chronic renal disease	

CASE STUDIES

Case 1

A 68-year-old man with congestive heart failure (CHF) is being treated with a combination of diet and diuretics. He returns from a trip to New Orleans complaining of difficulty breathing and swollen ankles. He is admitted to the coronary care unit for observation and treatment. Auscultation reveals bilateral inspiratory crackles in the lung bases. His respiratory rate is 28 breaths/min, and his heart rate is 110 beats/min with arrhythmias.

39. Patients with CHF are usually placed on what special type of diet? Why?

40. Diuretics commonly cause loss of what specific electrolyte that affects cardiac function? How will this electrolyte be replaced in the hospital? The home?

   A. Electrolyte:_____

   B. Hospital replacement:_____

   C. Home replacement:_____

41. As a respiratory therapist, what action will you take to further assess cardiopulmonary status? What is likely to be your initial treatment of this patient?

42. What is the cause of this patient's lung crackles?

Copyright © 2025, Elsevier, Inc. All rights reserved.

A 68-year-old homeless alcoholic is found in respiratory distress by the paramedics and brought to your emergency department. The patient is malnourished. Auscultation reveals bilateral inspiratory crackles in the lung bases. His respiratory rate is 28 breaths/min with a heart rate of 110 beats/min. Hint: Look at the section on Starling equilibrium. We'll get back to these two cases again and again because pulmonary edema is such a common clinical problem; Chapter 29 is devoted to this topic. Now is a good time to get your feet wet in the area of flooded lungs.

43. What protein accounts for the high osmotic pressure of plasma? Why is this patient lacking this substance?

_____

44. Explain why this patient has crackles.

45. As a respiratory therapist, what action will you take to further assess cardiopulmonary status? What is likely to be your initial treatment of this patient?

MATHEMATICS

46. Albuterol is prepared in a 5% solution (weight/volume). How many grams of albuterol are dissolved in 100 ml to make this solution?

Formula _____

Solution _____

Answer _____

47. Respiratory therapists do not usually administer 100 ml of drugs to their patients. Instead, they give 1 ml or less. How many milligrams of albuterol would be found in 1 ml of the 5% solution in question 46?

Formula _____

Solution _____

Answer _____

48. After drawing up 1 ml of a 5% solution of albuterol into a syringe, the respiratory therapist places the bronchodilator into a nebulizer along with 2 ml of saline for dilution. The total solution is now 3 ml in the nebulizer. What is the new concentration of the drug?

Formula _____

Solution _____

Answer _____

Copyright © 2025, Elsevier, Inc. All rights reserved.

Circle the best answer for each of the following multiple-choice questions.

49. A patient with severe hypokalemia is receiving an intravenous infusion of potassium to correct this serious disorder. What should you monitor?
    A. SpO_2
    B. Respiratory frequency
    C. Mental status
    D. ECG rhythm

50. Which of the following signs and symptoms would you expect to observe in a patient with hypokalemia?
    1. Metabolic acid-base disturbance
    2. Muscle spasms and tetany
    3. ECG abnormality
       A. 1 only
       B. 1 and 2 only
       C. 1 and 3 only
       D. 2 and 3 only

51. Which of the following would not be consistent with administration of a large amount of IV fluid?
    A. increased pulmonary vascular markings on the chest x-ray.
    B. presence of crackles on auscultation.
    C. increased urine output.
    D. increased hematocrit.

52. A respiratory therapist delivers isotonic saline to a patient via nebulizer. What concentration of saline is the therapist delivering?
    A. 0.0%
    B. 0.45%
    C. 0.90%
    D. 1.0%

FOOD FOR THOUGHT

A medical student asked a respiratory therapist if the saline in his nebulizer treatment would hurt her patient, who was on sodium restriction for his heart. "No problem," said the RT. Use this scenario to answer the following question.

53. What happens to cells in the presence of a hypertonic solution?

    _____

54. What happens to cells in the presence of a hypotonic solution?

    _____

55. What is the name for the movement of water across a semipermeable membrane?

    _____

Copyright © 2025, Elsevier, Inc. All rights reserved.

14 Acid-Base Balance

14

WORD WIZARD

Match the following terms to their definitions.

Terms	Definitions
1. _____ Acidemia	A. Acid that can be excreted in gaseous form
2. _____ Volatile acid	B. Decreased hydrogen ion concentration in the blood
3. _____ Anion gap	C. Ventilation that results in decreased CO_2
4. _____ Hyperventilation	D. Respiratory processes resulting in increased hydrogen ions
5. _____ Metabolic acidosis	E. Nonvolatile acid representing the by-product of protein catabolism
6. _____ Alkalemia	F. Abnormal ventilator pattern in response to metabolic acidosis
7. _____ Kussmaul breathing	G. Nonrespiratory processes resulting in decreased hydrogen ions
8. _____ Hypoventilation	H. Difference between electrolyte concentrations
9. _____ Fixed acid	I. Respiratory processes resulting in decreased hydrogen ions
10. _____ Respiratory alkalosis	J. Increased hydrogen ion concentration in the blood
11. _____ Metabolic alkalosis	K. Nonrespiratory processes resulting in increased hydrogen ions
12. _____ Standard bicarbonate (HCO_3^-)	L. Chemical substance that minimizes fluctuations in pH
13. _____ Base excess	M. Plasma concentration of HCO_3^- corrected to a normal CO_2
14. _____ Respiratory acidosis	N. Difference between normal and actual buffers available
15. _____ Buffer	O. Ventilation that results in increased CO_2

WHERE HAS ALL THE ACID GONE?

16. Draw a diagram of the process called isohydric buffering.

67

Copyright © 2025, Elsevier, Inc. All rights reserved.

17. Explain how the lungs can compensate for increased production of fixed acids.

18. Buffers are composed of what two components? _____
_____

19. What happens when you add the acid hydrogen chloride to the base sodium bicarbonate?

20. What does ventilation remove from the body to help eliminate acid? Support your answer with information from the text.

21. Why are buffers in the kidney essential for the secretion of excess hydrogen ions?

BALANCING ACT

22. List the normal range of values for pH, $PaCO_2$, and HCO_3^-. (You MUST memorize these values!)

	Low Normal	High Normal
A. pH		
B. $PaCO_2$		
C. HCO_3^-		

Copyright © 2025, Elsevier, Inc. All rights reserved.

23. Write out the Henderson-Hasselbalch equation.

24. Complete the primary acid-base and compensation chart below.

	Disorder	Primary Defect	Compensation
A.	Respiratory acidosis		
B.	Respiratory alkalosis		
C.	Metabolic acidosis		
D.	Metabolic alkalosis		

25. What is the "rule of thumb" for determining the expected increase in HCO_3^- for any acute increase in CO_2?

26. How much will HCO_3^- increase with a chronic increase in CO_2?

THE METHOD

There is a simple four-step method for interpreting blood gas values.

Step 1: Determine the pH first.
Step 2: Evaluate respiratory status ($PaCO_2$) to see if it agrees with the pH.
Step 3: Evaluate metabolic status (HCO_3^-) to see if it agrees.
Step 4: Evaluate compensation.

Interpret the following blood gas results.

27. pH   7.34
    $PaCO_2$ 60 mm Hg
    HCO_3^- 31 mEq/L

69

Copyright © 2025, Elsevier, Inc. All rights reserved.

28. pH   7.36
    $PaCO_2$ 60 mm Hg
    HCO_3^- 33 mEq/L

Stop right there! We're going to continue interpreting blood gas results in the case studies and board examination review questions, but you can see how the HCO_3^- will be creeping up as the CO_2 rises and the pH returns to low normal to compensate.

THE ANION GAP

29. Name the three common causes of anion gap metabolic acidosis.

    A. _____

    B. _____

    C. _____

30. What are the signs of respiratory compensation for metabolic acidosis?

31. What are the neurologic symptoms of severe acidosis?

    _____

MATHEMATICS

32. Calculate the new HCO_3^- (assume 24 mEq/L as the starting point) level for an acutely elevated $PaCO_2$ of 70 mm Hg (assume it started at 40 mm Hg).

    Formula _____

    Solution _____

    Answer _____

33. Calculate the new HCO_3^- (assume 24 mEq/L as the starting point) level for a *chronically* elevated $PaCO_2$ of 70 mm Hg (assume it started at 40 mm Hg).

    Formula _____

    Solution _____

    Answer _____

34. Calculate pH if HCO_3^- is 30 mEq/L and $PaCO_2$ is 40 mm Hg.

    Formula _____

    Solution _____

    Answer _____

35. Calculate pH if HCO_3^- is 24 mEq/L and $PaCO_2$ is 40 mm Hg.

    Formula _____

    Solution _____

    Answer _____

Copyright © 2025, Elsevier, Inc. All rights reserved.

36. Calculate pH if HCO$_3^-$ is 24 mEq/L and PaCO$_2$ is 60 mm Hg.

Formula _____

Solution _____

Answer _____

37. Calculate anion gap if Na$^+$ is 144 mEq/ml, Cl$^-$ is 100 mEq/ml, and HCO$_3^-$ is 22 mEq/ml.

Formula _____

Solution _____

Answer _____

38. Calculate anion gap if Na$^+$ is 135 mEq/ml, Cl$^-$ is 105 mEq/ml, and HCO$_3^-$ is 26 mEq/ml.

Formula _____

Solution _____

Answer _____

CASE STUDIES

The following case studies will systematically take you through the major acid-base disorders. Let's start with some simple, acute states and move into the compensated ones. Remember to evaluate using the four-step process.

Case 1

Mrs. Mary Maladie was depressed and took too much diazepam (Valium). She is found *shortly* thereafter in a coma breathing slowly and shallowly. ABG results reveal pH of 7.28, PaCO$_2$ of 60 mm Hg, and HCO$_3^-$ of 26 mEq/L.

39. How would you interpret this ABG? _____

_____

40. What is the primary cause of the disorder? _____

_____

Case 2

Mrs. M's husband, Jim, is very worried about her condition. He complains of dizziness and tingling in his hands. ABG results reveal pH of 7.58, PaCO$_2$ of 25 mm Hg, and HCO$_3^-$ of 23 mEq/L.

41. How would you interpret this ABG? _____

42. What is the primary cause of the disorder? _____

Copyright © 2025, Elsevier, Inc. All rights reserved.

Case 3

The couple's young son, Billy, has been sick with the stomach flu. ABG results reveal pH of 7.60, $PaCO_2$ of 40 mm Hg, and HCO_3^- of 38 mEq/L.

43. How would you interpret this ABG? _____

44. What is the primary cause of the disorder? _____

Case 4

The couple's diabetic teenage daughter, Lizzy, has not been taking her insulin. ABG results reveal pH of 7.25, $PaCO_2$ of 40 mm Hg, and HCO_3^- of 17 mEq/L.

45. How would you interpret this ABG? _____

46. What is the primary cause of the disorder? _____
Of course, blood gases, like children, don't stay simple for long. Partial or complete compensation may occur.

Case 5

Grandpa Maladie has smoked for years, and now he has COPD. ABG results reveal pH of 7.37, $PaCO_2$ of 50 mm Hg, and HCO_3^- of 28 mEq/L.

47. How would you interpret this ABG? _____

48. What is the source of compensation? _____

Case 6

As soon as Lizzy Maladie's brain realizes the acute nature of her illness (Case 4), compensation begins. ABG results now reveal pH of 7.35, $PaCO_2$ of 25 mm Hg, and HCO_3^- of 13 mEq/L.

49. How would you interpret this ABG? _____

50. What is the source of compensation? _____

Case 7

Grandma Maladie has congestive heart failure. She takes furosemide (Lasix) to reduce extra water in her body. ABG results now reveal pH of 7.46, $PaCO_2$ of 45 mm Hg, and HCO_3^- of 31 mEq/L.

51. How would you interpret this ABG? _____

52. What is a possible cause of the primary disorder? _____

WHAT DOES THE NBRC SAY?

Circle the best answer to the following multiple choice questions.

53. A 17-year-old girl is brought to the emergency department by paramedics. Her mother states she is a diabetic. Room air ABGs reveal the following:

pH	7.26
$PaCO_2$	16 mm Hg
HCO_3^-	8 mEq/L
PaO_2	110 mm Hg

Copyright © 2025, Elsevier, Inc. All rights reserved.

This information indicates which of the following?
1. Partly compensated metabolic acidosis is present.
2. This PaO_2 is not possible on room air.
3. Respiratory alkalosis is present.
   A. 1 only
   B. 3 only
   C. 1 and 2 only
   D. 1 and 3 only

54. Interpret the following ABG results:

F_iO_2	0.21
pH	7.36
$PaCO_2$	37 mm Hg
HCO_3^-	22 mEq/L
PaO_2	95 mm Hg

   A. Acute respiratory alkalosis
   B. Acute metabolic alkalosis
   C. Compensated respiratory alkalosis
   D. Normal ABG

55. During CPR, blood gases are drawn. The results are as follows:

F_iO_2	1.0
pH	7.15
$PaCO_2$	55 mm Hg
HCO_3^-	12 mEq/L
PaO_2	210 mm Hg

   What action should be taken to correct the acid-base abnormality shown here?
   A. Increase the rate of ventilation.
   B. Decrease the F_iO_2.
   C. Administer sodium bicarbonate intravenously.
   D. Add positive end-expiratory pressure (PEEP) to the ventilation system.

56. The results of an arterial blood gas measurement are as follows:

F_iO_2	0.21
pH	7.55
$PaCO_2$	25 mm Hg
HCO_3^-	24 mEq/L
PaO_2	105 mm Hg

   These data indicate which of the following?
   A. Metabolic acidosis
   B. Metabolic alkalosis
   C. Uncompensated hyperventilation
   D. Uncompensated hypoventilation

57. A 72-year-old man with a history of renal failure is seen in the emergency department. The respiratory therapist notes that the patient is taking 28 very deep breaths per minute. Which of the following accurately describes this breathing pattern?
   A. Cheyne-Stokes breathing
   B. Ataxic breathing
   C. Kussmaul breathing
   D. Eupneic breathing

Copyright © 2025, Elsevier, Inc. All rights reserved.

Blood gas disorders can get really complicated at times. In some cases, a patient will have one disorder superimposed on another.

Grandpa Maladie, discussed in Case 5, acquired a lung infection after visiting his daughter in the hospital. ABG results now reveal pH of 7.46 (pH previously 7.37), $PaCO_2$ of 55 mm Hg (previously 50 mm Hg), PaO_2 of 57 mm Hg, and HCO_3^- of 38 mEq/L (previously 28 mEq/L).

58. How would you interpret this ABG?

59. Why did the blood gas values change from those in the case?

Copyright © 2025, Elsevier, Inc. All rights reserved.

15 Regulation of Breathing

1. What is the term used to describes when there is no breathing at all?

2. What reflexes may be stimulated during airway suctioning or bronchoscopy?

3. What do apneustic center impulses do?

4. What barrier prevents many substances from entering the cerebrospinal fluid?

5. What center in the pons helps increase rate and control depth of ventilation and inspiratory time?

6. What receptors responds to changes in O_2 and pH to signal the need to breathe?

Copyright © 2025, Elsevier, Inc. All rights reserved.

7. Label the parts of these central controlling bodies.

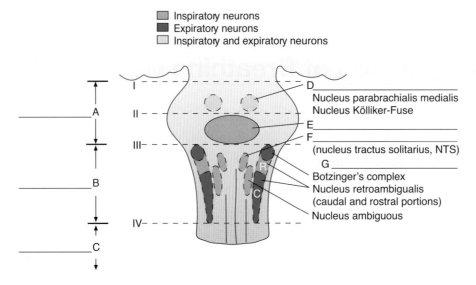

☐ Inspiratory neurons
■ Expiratory neurons
☐ Inspiratory and expiratory neurons

D_____
Nucleus parabrachialis medialis
Nucleus Kölliker-Fuse
E_____
F_____
(nucleus tractus solitarius, NTS)
G _____
Botzinger's complex
Nucleus retroambigualis
(caudal and rostral portions)
Nucleus ambiguous

8. Briefly explain the role of the two primary respiratory groups in the medulla.

9. Compare and contrast the apneustic and pneumotaxic centers in the pons.

10. What diseases or conditions might affect the performance of the brainstem's respiratory controllers?

AUTOMATIC PILOT

Finish the following chart by filling in the correct terms.

	REFLEX	STIMULUS	RESPONSE	LOCATION
11.	Hering-Breuer			
12.	Deflation			
13.	Head			
14.	Vagovagal			
15.	C fiber			
16.	Proprioceptors			

Copyright © 2025, Elsevier, Inc. All rights reserved.

17. Explain the process that allows CO_2 to stimulate the central receptors.

18. Describe the stimulating effects of CO_2 on the receptors in terms of the immediate response to increased CO_2 in the blood. What happens when this goes on for 1 or 2 days?

19. Describe the peripheral receptor response to decreased arterial O_2 levels. What do the receptors actually respond to when O_2 levels drop?

20. What specific range of PaO_2 values causes the greatest response when CO_2 and pH are normal?

21. How does altitude modify the receptor's response to hypoxemia?

22. Describe the peripheral receptor response to increased arterial CO_2 and H^+ ions. How is it different from the central chemoreceptor response?

23. What concentration of O_2 is usually given to chronically hypercapnic patients?

24. What is the best way to monitor oxygenation in these patients?

Copyright © 2025, Elsevier, Inc. All rights reserved.

25. Why do low concentrations of O_2 usually result in adequate improvement?

26. Describe Cheyne-Stokes breathing (use words or draw a picture). State two important causes of this distinctive pattern.

27. How does Biot breathing differ from Cheyne-Stokes in terms of pattern and origin?

28. Describe apneustic breathing. What does this pattern indicate?

29. What are the two central neurogenic breathing patterns? State three events that could cause these patterns.

CASE STUDIES

Case 1

Your patient rode his motorcycle without a helmet. He sustained a closed head injury during a crash that resulted in a subdural hematoma. The paramedics endotracheally intubated him and transported him to the emergency department.

30. Hyperventilation may lower the intracranial pressure of a patient with traumatic brain injury. What rules would you follow if you decide to do this procedure?
    A. When:
    B. Lowest safe CO_2 value:
    C. Length of time you can safely hyperventilate:

    _____

31. Why is lowering the CO_2 level controversial in traumatic brain injury?

Copyright © 2025, Elsevier, Inc. All rights reserved.

Case 2

Grandpa Charlie, a COPD patient, is back in the hospital. He became short of breath at home, and his family increased his O_2 from 2 to 6 L/min. When he arrives at the hospital, he is somnolent and difficult to arouse. ABG results reveal that pH is 7.25, $PaCO_2$ is 75 mm Hg, PaO_2 is 90 mm Hg, and HCO_3^- level is 37 mEq/L on 6 L/min by nasal cannula.

32. What changes should you make in the patient's therapy? Why?

33. What target PaO_2 would be more appropriate for this patient? (Consider the PO_2 at which the receptors kick in.)

WHAT DOES THE NBRC SAY?

Circle the best answer for each of the following multiple choice questions.

34. A patient who has had COPD for many years is admitted for an acute episode of dyspnea. Arterial blood gas measured in the patient breathing room air gives these results:

pH	7.50
$PaCO_2$	48 mm Hg
PaO_2	44 mm Hg
HCO_3^-	36 mEq/L
SaO_2	84%

    What therapy do you recommend at this time?
    A. 28% Venturi mask
    B. 35% Venturi mask
    C. Nasal cannula delivering O_2 at 5 L/min
    D. Simple mask delivering O_2 at 10 L/min

35. A cooperative elderly patient with chronic asthma is examined at her pulmonologist's office. You observe the following findings:

Pulse	94 beats/min
RR	28 breaths/min
Temperature	36.5°C
BP	135/90 mm Hg
F_iO_2	0.21
pH	7.33
$PaCO_2$	70 mm Hg
PaO_2	35 mm Hg
HCO_3^-	34 mEq/L

    What action would you take at this time?
    A. Administer bronchodilator therapy via MDI and holding chamber.
    B. Administer O_2 via cannula at 2 L/min.
    C. Administer O_2 via cannula at 6 L/min.
    D. Administer O_2 via nonrebreathing mask.

Copyright © 2025, Elsevier, Inc. All rights reserved.

36. A patient with COPD and a history of hypercapnia is receiving O_2 via simple mask at 10 L/min in the recovery room following admission for pneumonia. Upon transfer to the medical floor, he is noted to be increasingly drowsy and difficult to arouse. The nurse requests that you give him a breathing treatment with a bronchodilator. The most appropriate action would be to
   A. administer the breathing treatment as requested.
   B. obtain an arterial blood gas sample.
   C. change the O_2 to 2 L/min via nasal cannula.
   D. change the O_2 to 40% via Venturi mask.

37. A patient is being mechanically ventilated following craniotomy. During a suctioning procedure, the intracranial pressure monitor shows a sudden increase in intracranial pressure. The patient becomes restless and agitated. What is the most appropriate immediate action for the respiratory therapist in this situation?
   A. Increase the F_iO_2 on the ventilator to deliver 100% O_2.
   B. Recommend administration of a sedative.
   C. Increase rate and volume of ventilation with a resuscitation bag.
   D. Ask the registered nurse to page the physician "STAT."

EXPERIMENT

This exercise may seem simple, but it will help you understand control of breathing. It's even better if you have a pulse oximeter.
- Put the oximeter probe on your finger.
- Breathe normally.
- Now inhale deeply and hold your breath.
- Time how long you can hold your breath.
- Next, inhale and exhale deeply several times. Fill your lungs and time how long you can hold your breath. (Remember to be seated and have a partner.)
- Answer the following questions.

38. How long could you hold your breath the first time? _____ What about the second

   try? _____

39. What were the pulse oximetry readings before _____, during _____, and at the end of breath holding?

40. Compare the results and explain the differences in the breath-holding time and why you had to breathe. What is the meaning of the pulse oximetry readings?

SUMMARY CHECKLIST

41. What groups of neurons in the medulla generate the basic cyclic breathing pattern?

42. Where are the peripheral chemoreceptors located that respond to arterial [H+]?

Copyright © 2025, Elsevier, Inc. All rights reserved.

43. What increases the sensitivity of chemoreceptors to a given arterial pH?

44. What is the primary stimulus for breathing in healthy individuals?

45. The breathing of patients with chronic hypercapnia is driven more by _____ stimulus than in patients with normal acid-base status.

46. _____ therapy is associated with acute arterial CO_2 retention in patients with chronic

_____.

FOOD FOR THOUGHT

47. Why do we measure patients' respiratory rates without telling them we are doing it?

48. Name as many factors as you can that involve the higher brain centers increasing the rate of ventilation.

49. An astronomy student goes to the volcano observatory (elevation 11,000 feet) for his first clinical assignment. What is likely to happen to his breathing pattern as he goes higher up the mountain? What causes this to happen?

50. What would happen over the next 24 hours and why?

Copyright © 2025, Elsevier, Inc. All rights reserved.

16 Bedside Assessment of the Patient

WORD WIZARD

Match the following terms to their definitions as they apply to respiratory care.

Definitions		Terms
1. _____	Musical inspiratory or expiratory sound associated with asthma	A. Angina
2. _____	Difficulty breathing when lying supine	B. Barrel chest
3. _____	Shape of thorax associated with emphysema	C. Bradycardia
4. _____	Chest pain typical of acute coronary syndromes	D. Breathlessness
5. _____	Physical wasting associated with chronic lung disease	E. Cachexia
6. _____	Blood pressure that is too low	F. Crackles
7. _____	The sitting position that emphysema patients use when they are in trouble	G. Cyanosis
8. _____	Drop in blood pressure on inhalation associated with asthma and hyperinflation	H. Dyspnea
9. _____	Inspiratory sound associated with atelectasis, pneumonia, and fibrosis	I. Febrile
10. _____	Upper airway sound that may indicate life-threatening obstruction	J. Orthopnea
11. _____	Soft tissue sucking in around ribs and neck when a patient has severe distress	K. Pulse deficit
12. _____	Dizziness associated with drop in blood pressure	L. Pulse pressure
13. _____	A rapid heart rate that may indicate a low blood oxygen level	M. Pulsus paradoxus
14. _____	Presence of a fever	N. Retractions
15. _____	Difference between systolic and diastolic blood pressure	O. Shock
16. _____	A slow heart rate that may result in poor perfusion of tissues	P. Stridor
17. _____	Bluish discoloration of skin often associated with hypoxemia	Q. Syncope
18. _____	Heart rate auscultated in chest is different than pulse rate felt in arm	R. Tachycardia
19. _____	Difficulty breathing	S. Tripoding
20. _____	Sensation of suffocation	T. Wheezes

Copyright © 2025, Elsevier, Inc. All rights reserved.

21. What information would you gather before entering the patient's room?

22. Describe how to *start* the ideal interview. Be sure to discuss space, privacy, and introductions.

A. Space: _____

B. Privacy: _____

C. Introductions: _____

23. Circle the *best approach* from each set of choices in the following list:
    A1. "Hi, Bob, good morning."
    A2. "Good morning, Mr. Johnson."

    B1. Stand at the foot of the bed.
    B2. Sit in a chair at the bedside.

    C1. Make room for your notes on the bedside table.
    C2. Keep your clipboard on your lap.

    D1. "Do you need anything right now?"
    D2. "I'll tell your nurse to check on you."

    E1. "I'll be back to see you in one hour."
    E2. "I'll return in a while to check on you."

24. Circle the best approach from each set of choices in following list:
    A1. "What are you coughing up?"
    A2. "You didn't cough up blood, did you?"

    B1. "I understand you don't like your breathing treatments."
    B2. "Why don't you like these treatments?"

    C1. "How is your breathing today?"
    C2. "Is your breathing better today?"

25. When are "closed" questions most useful? Give an example.

SIGNS AND SYMPTOMS OF CARDIOPULMONARY DISEASE

26. Describe the dyspnea (Borg) scale. List several reasons why this scale would be useful.

Copyright © 2025, Elsevier, Inc. All rights reserved.

27. How else can you identify the degree of dyspnea a patient feels? Explain the difference between dyspnea and breathlessness.

28. What are the possible causes of these common types of cough?

	Cough	Cause(s)
A.	Dry	
B.	Loose, productive	
C.	Acute, self-limiting	
D.	Chronic	

29. What is the difference between mucus and sputum?

30. What are the three characteristics of sputum that should be documented and reported to the physician and other members of the health care team?

_____

_____

_____

31. What is the most serious kind of nonpleuritic chest pain?

_____

_____

32. How does pleuritic chest pain differ from nonpleuritic pain?

33. Significant elevation of temperature will have what result on metabolic rate, oxygen consumption, carbon dioxide production, and breathing pattern?

_____

_____

Copyright © 2025, Elsevier, Inc. All rights reserved.

34. Along with fever, what are two signs that are highly suggestive of respiratory infection?

    A. _____

    B. _____

35. What do the initials "CC" and "HPI" stand for? List at least five important areas described in the HPI.

    A. CC = _____

    B. HPI = _____

       1. _____

       2. _____

       3. _____

       4. _____

       5. _____

36. What do the initials "PMH" stand for? List at least five important areas described in the PMH.

    A. PMH = _____

       1. _____

       2. _____

       3. _____

       4. _____

       5. _____

37. Describe the significance of the findings for each of the areas of general appearance listed below.

	FINDING	SIGNIFICANCE
1.	Weak, emaciated, and diaphoretic	
2.	Appears anxious	
3.	Sitting up, leaning with arms on table	

38. What does the phrase "oriented × 4" mean?

    _____

39. Compare and contrast the terms "lethargic" and "obtunded."

Copyright © 2025, Elsevier, Inc. All rights reserved.

40. What is the difference between a "stuporous" patient and a "comatose" patient?

41. What is the first thing a respiratory therapist should evaluate in cases of a decreased level of consciousness?

_____

VITAL INFORMATION

42. Fill in the correct normal values (or terms) for an adult in the chart below.

	SIGN	AVERAGE NORMAL	LOWEST NORMAL	HIGHEST NORMAL
A.	Temperature			
B.	Heart rate			
C.	Respiratory rate			
D.	Systolic blood pressure			
E.	Diastolic blood pressure			

43. Match these terms to their definitions.

Terms	Definitions
A. Bruits	1. Palpable vibrations in pulse
B. Amplitude	2. Strength of pulse
C. Paradoxical pulse	3. Drop in amplitude with inspiration
D. Pulsus alternans	4. Alternating strong and weak pulses

44. Match these respiratory patterns to their definitions.

Patterns	Definitions
A. Tachypnea	1. Difficulty breathing in a supine position
B. Eupnea	2. Abnormally low respiratory rate
C. Platypnea	3. Deep breathing
D. Hyperpnea	4. Normal breathing pattern
E. Bradypnea	5. Abnormally high respiratory rate
	6. Labored breathing in an upright position

45. How can you prevent patients from becoming aware (and consciously altering their breathing) that you are taking their respiratory rate?

Copyright © 2025, Elsevier, Inc. All rights reserved.

46. What does it mean when patients show a larger (>10 mm Hg) decrease in pulse strength during spontaneous inspiration?

47. Write a description for the following abnormal chest shapes.

Abnormal chest shape	Description
A. Barrel	_____
B. Kyphosis	_____
C. Kyphoscoliosis	_____
D. Pectus carinatum	_____
E. Pectus excavatum	_____
F. Scoliosis	_____

48. Explain the difference between vocal and tactile fremitus.

49. Describe the difference between fremitus in emphysema and in pneumonia.

50. How does subcutaneous emphysema form? What is the feeling of air under the skin called?

51. Complete the following chart by identifying the percussion notes for the conditions.

Condition	Percussion Note
A. Emphysema	_____
B. Atelectasis	_____
C. Pleural effusion	_____
D. Pneumothorax	_____
E. Pneumonia	_____

Copyright © 2025, Elsevier, Inc. All rights reserved.

52. What are the limitations of percussion? What can't you palpate?_____

_____

53. Fill in the chart below with descriptions of your favorite breath sounds.

	BREATH SOUND	PITCH	INTENSITY	LOCATION
A.	Vesicular			
B.	Bronchial			
C.	Bronchovesicular			

54. Compare the mechanisms and causes of coarse, low-pitched crackles and fine, end-inspiratory crackles.

55. Contrast monophonic and polyphonic wheezes in terms of mechanisms, phase of ventilation, and conditions that produce these different musical sounds.

56. How do you test for capillary refill? What is a normal capillary refill time?

57. Where should you check for edema caused by heart failure? Why? _____

_____

58. Answer the following questions about cyanosis.

A. What is the specific cause of cyanosis? _____

_____

B. What is peripheral cyanosis? _____

_____

C. What is the main cause of peripheral cyanosis? _____

_____

Copyright © 2025, Elsevier, Inc. All rights reserved.

Chapter **16** **Bedside Assessment of the Patient**

Case 1

An alert 67-year-old male is admitted for dyspnea and hemoptysis. While interviewing the patient you discover that he has been coughing up small amounts of thick, blood-streaked mucus several times per day for the last few days. He has a history of 100 pack-years of cigarette smoking. Physical examination reveals a barrel chest, use of accessory muscles, and digital clubbing.

59. The patient's history and chest configuration suggest what primary pulmonary disorder?

_____

_____

60. Along with enlargement of the ends of the fingers, what sign helps you recognize clubbing?

_____

_____

61. What does the presence of clubbing suggest in this case?

_____

_____

Case 2

A 47-year-old female is admitted for a systemic infection 3 days after cutting herself in the kitchen while preparing some chicken. She complains of dyspnea and has a fever. Her vital signs are pulse 110 beats/min, respiratory rate 28 breaths/min, and blood pressure 76/58 mm Hg. The nurse's notes reveal that the patient was alert on admission, but she is now confused and anxious. Her extremities are warm, and capillary refill is normal.

62. Why do you think the patient's mental status has deteriorated?

63. What other "vital sign" should be evaluated? _____

_____

64. Which abnormal vital sign has the most clinical significance in this case?

_____

_____

Copyright © 2025, Elsevier, Inc. All rights reserved.

65. There are vibrations on exhalation over the upper chest. What action should be taken at this time?
    A. The patient should be given a bronchodilator.
    B. The patient should be suctioned.
    C. The patient should be given supplemental oxygen.
    D. The patient should be placed on mechanical ventilation.

66. A patient's medical record indicates that he has orthopnea. Which of the following best describes this condition?
    A. Difficulty breathing at night
    B. Difficulty breathing when upright
    C. Difficulty breathing on exertion
    D. Difficulty breathing when lying down

67. A child is brought to the emergency department for severe respiratory distress. Upon entering the room, the RT hears a high-pitched sound when the child inhales. This is most likely
    A. wheezing.
    B. stridor.
    C. rhonchi.
    D. crackles.

68. An RT is asked to evaluate a patient for oxygen therapy. She notices that the patient is sleepy but arouses when questioned. This level of consciousness is best described as
    A. confused.
    B. obtunded.
    C. stuporous.
    D. lethargic.

69. During an interview, the patient states he has been coughing up thick, foul-smelling sputum. This finding is most consistent with
    A. a bacterial infection of the lung.
    B. a diagnosis of lung cancer.
    C. obstructive lung disease.
    D. pulmonary tuberculosis.

70. An RT is inspecting the chest of a child with respiratory distress. The practitioner notes that the child has a large concave depression of the sternum. This finding should be documented as
    A. barrel chest.
    B. pectus carinatum.
    C. pectus excavatum.
    D. kyphoscoliosis.

Copyright © 2025, Elsevier, Inc. All rights reserved.

17 Interpreting Clinical and Laboratory Data

LAB TESTS

1. What may a large elevation in white blood cell (WBC) count suggest?

   A. _____

   B. _____

   C. _____

2. List three common causes of low WBC count.

   A. _____

   B. _____

   C. _____

3. What specific type of WBC is elevated in bacterial pneumonia? Viral pneumonia?

   A. Bacterial: _____

   B. Viral: _____

4. Which WBCs are involved in problems such as allergic asthma?

5. What term describes a low red blood cell (RBC) count? What is the treatment for this disorder?

   A. Term: _____

   B. Treatment: _____

   _____

6. What is a normal hemoglobin level, and why are RTs especially interested in hemoglobin levels?

   A. Normal: _____

   B. Respiratory role: _____

   _____

7. What blood abnormality is caused by chronic hypoxemia? _____

   _____

Copyright © 2025, Elsevier, Inc. All rights reserved.

8. Before performing an arterial blood gas (ABG), you would be wise to check which two *specific* laboratory values?

   A. Blood count _____

   B. Blood chemistry test _____

9. What is the normal range for serum potassium?

   _____

10. Why is potassium of particular interest in patients being weaned from mechanical ventilation?

11. Give at least one clinical example of how a patient develops a very high or very low potassium level.

    A. Hyperkalemia _____

    B. Hypokalemia _____

12. What value on the venous chemistry panel represents bicarbonate?

    _____

13. Low chloride levels occur for what two primary reasons?

    A. _____

    B. _____

14. Why is the chloride level in sweat so important? What is the critical value?

    A. Importance: _____

    B. Value: _____

15. What other test is indicated when a chemistry panel shows an abnormal anion gap?

    _____

16. What are the two tests that together indicate renal function?

    _____

17. Name the two common liver enzymes that might be elevated in patients with hepatitis.

    A. _____

    B. _____

18. CPK is an example of an enzyme that can show you specific injury to brain, lungs, heart, or muscles. Describe the three types of CPK and what they mean.

    A. CPK-BB _____

    B. CPK-MM _____

    C. CPK-MB _____

Copyright © 2025, Elsevier, Inc. All rights reserved.

Chapter **17** **Interpreting Clinical and Laboratory Data**

19. Discuss troponin I and explain why it would be important in emergency medicine.

20. Another interesting chemical can tell you if the patient has heart failure rather than a heart attack. What does BNP stand for and how do we use this test?

    A. BNP = _____

    B. What does it show us? _____

    C. Name another condition that can elevate BNP. _____

21. What is PT?

    A. Full name _____

    B. When is it used? _____

22. What is PTT?

    A. Full name _____

    B. When is it used? _____

    C. Explain the difference in the two tests.

    D. Name medications associated with PTT.

23. Explain the D-dimer test and how it is useful to respiratory therapists.

24. What blood cell is vital to clotting, and what is its normal value?

Copyright © 2025, Elsevier, Inc. All rights reserved.

25. Why would the laboratory reject your sputum specimen? Give specific reasons and include numerical values.

A. Pus _____

B. Epithelial cells_____

How can you improve the quality?

_____

_____

26. What is the purpose of growing the bacteria on a culture plate?

CASE STUDIES

Case 1

A patient presents in the emergency department complaining of shortness of breath, fever, and productive cough. A chest radiograph reveals pneumonia in the right lower lobe.

27. What blood test is indicated?

_____

28. What specific finding would suggest bacterial pneumonia?

_____

29. What would you like to do about the sputum?

Case 2

A 60-year-old, two-pack-per-day smoker has a complete blood count ordered, and his WBC count is 9000. His hematocrit is 60%, and his hemoglobin is 20 g/dL.

30. What is the name for this elevation of red blood cells?

_____

31. What respiratory problem is indicated by the high hematocrit and hemoglobin?

_____

WHAT DOES THE NBRC SAY?

32. Sputum culture and sensitivity would be indicated for which of the following conditions?
    A. ST segment elevation
    B. Pleural effusion
    C. Pneumothorax
    D. Bronchitis

95

Copyright © 2025, Elsevier, Inc. All rights reserved.

33. A patient presents in the emergency department with vomiting. Blood gas results reveal metabolic alkalosis. Based on this information, you would also suggest
    A. a STAT chest radiograph.
    B. an electrolyte analysis.
    C. a complete blood count.
    D. clotting time.

34. A sputum culture that is sent to the lab is likely to be rejected as saliva if
    A. fewer than 25 epithelial cells are present.
    B. fewer than 25 pus cells are present.
    C. more than 25 epithelial cells are present.
    D. more than 25 pus cells are present.

FOOD FOR THOUGHT

35. A young adult male patient presents with symptoms of hypoxemia and signs of pneumonia. What are several possible reasons the WBC count is severely depressed?

Copyright © 2025, Elsevier, Inc. All rights reserved.

18 Interpreting the Electrocardiogram

ANATOMY OF THE IMPULSE-CONDUCTING SYSTEM OF THE HEART

Label the heart parts (1-9) and fill in the anatomical term for the conduction clues (10-17).

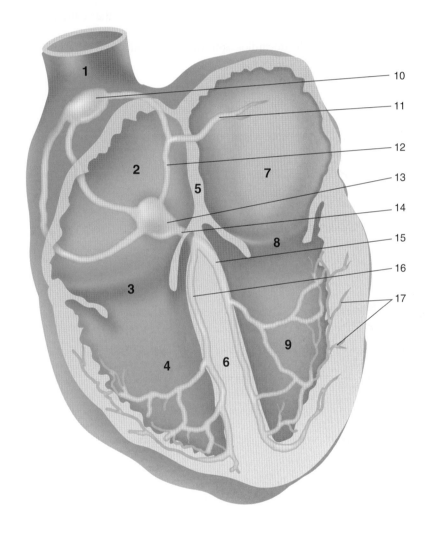

Copyright © 2025, Elsevier, Inc. All rights reserved.

Heart Parts	Conduction Clues

Heart Parts

1. _____

2. _____

3. _____

4. _____

5. _____

6. _____

7. _____

8. _____

9. _____

Conduction Clues

10. _____ Natural "pacemaker" of the heart

11. _____ Conducts impulses through the atria

12. _____ Carries impulses across the right atrium

13. _____ "Backup pacemaker"

14. _____ Bundle of cardiac fibers that conducts impulses that regulate the heartbeat

15. _____ Carries impulse to the left ventricle

16. _____ Carries impulse to the right ventricle

17. _____ Finger-like projections that penetrate the ventricles

18. Identify the normal configuration of electrocardiograph waves, segments, and intervals along with what they represent in the spaces below.

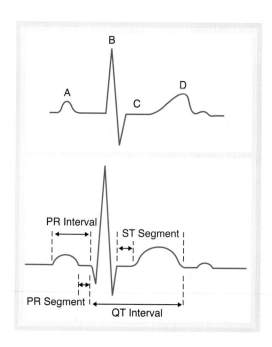

Wave, segment, and intervals

A. P wave

B. QRS complex

C. ST segment

D. T wave

Represents

_____

_____

_____

_____

Now answer the following questions about ECG waves.

19. Where is atrial repolarization?

_____

98

Copyright © 2025, Elsevier, Inc. All rights reserved.

20. What is the maximum duration of the P–R interval?

_____

21. What pathologic abnormality results in a depressed or elevated ST segment?

_____

MAKING MEASUREMENTS

22. What is the normal paper speed for an ECG?

_____

23. The time (horizontal axis) represented by one small box is _____ seconds and by one large box is _____ seconds.

24. One millivolt of electrical energy will produce a deflection of _____ small boxes or _____ large boxes.

Successful ECG interpretation begins with a systematic evaluation of the ECG.
Step 1: Evaluate the Rate

25. The number of QRS complexes in this 6-second strip is _____. Multiply by 10 to get a rate of _____.

26. There are _____ heavy lines between complex A and complex B; 300 divided by this number is _____. That's the average rate!

   Is every P wave followed by a QRS complex? That indicates a sinus rhythm!

27. If the rate is below 60 beats/min, it is called sinus _____.

28. If the rate is above 100 beats/min, it is called sinus _____.

Copyright © 2025, Elsevier, Inc. All rights reserved.

Step 2: Measure the P–R Interval

29. The time from the P wave to the QRS complex is _____ second(s).

30. What arrhythmia does this represent?

_____

Step 3: Evaluate the QRS Complex

31. The duration of the QRS complex is _____ second(s).

Step 4: Evaluate the T Wave

32. The T wave in pattern 1 is (circle one)

    upright

    inverted

Copyright © 2025, Elsevier, Inc. All rights reserved.

Step 5: Evaluate the ST Segment

33. The ST segment in pattern 4 is (circle one)

    elevated

    flat

    depressed

Step 6: Identify the RR Interval

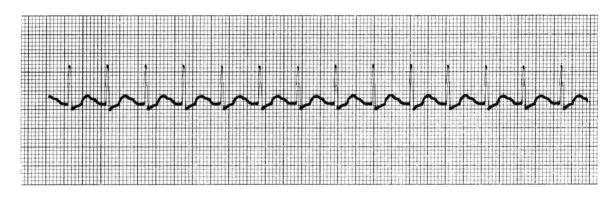

34. The RR interval in this pattern is (circle one)

    regular

    irregular

CASE STUDIES

Case 1

A student is suctioning a patient orally with a tonsil suction. The monitor shows sinus bradycardia. Blood pressure is falling. Alarms are sounding.

35. What should the student do?

36. What physiologic mechanism was responsible for the drop in rate?

Copyright © 2025, Elsevier, Inc. All rights reserved.

Case 2

A student is suctioning a patient via the endotracheal tube. The monitor shows sinus tachycardia with frequent premature ventricular contractions. Alarms are sounding. The patient is agitated.

37. What should this student do about the arrhythmias? _____

38. What physiologic mechanism was responsible for the increased rate and arrhythmias?

_____

Case 3

While performing a ventilator check on a patient in the coronary care unit, a student observes the rhythm on the monitor has changed from atrial fibrillation to ventricular fibrillation.

39. What should the student do first?

40. Name at least three responses indicated to treat this rhythm.

WHAT DOES THE NBRC SAY?

Circle the best answer.

41. An RT is suctioning a patient on a ventilator and observes the following rhythm on the monitor:

In regard to this pattern, the RT should
A. continue to suction the patient.
B. stop and administer 100% oxygen.
C. recommend atropine administration.
D. defibrillate the patient.

   Copyright © 2025, Elsevier, Inc. All rights reserved.

42. An RT is preparing to perform an arterial puncture when the following rhythm is observed on the monitor:

In regard to this pattern, the RT should
A. continue to suction the patient.
B. stop and administer 100% oxygen.
C. recommend atropine administration.
D. defibrillate the patient.

43. During a routine suctioning procedure, an RT notes the following rhythm on the cardiac monitor:

In regard to this pattern, the RT should
A. continue to suction the patient.
B. stop and administer 100% oxygen.
C. recommend atropine administration.
D. defibrillate the patient.

44. During a routine suctioning procedure, an RT notes the following rhythm on the cardiac monitor:

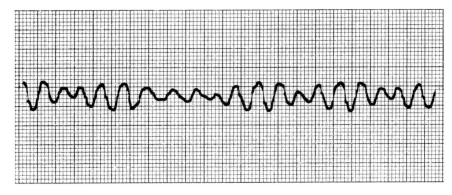

In regard to this pattern, the RT should
A. continue to suction the patient.
B. stop and administer 100% oxygen.
C. recommend atropine administration.
D. defibrillate the patient.

Copyright © 2025, Elsevier, Inc. All rights reserved.

45. A respiratory therapist is called to perform a STAT ECG on a patient with chest pain in the emergency department. Proper placement of chest lead V6 is the
   A. fourth intercostal space, left sternal margin.
   B. fourth intercostal space, right sternal margin.
   C. fifth intercostal space, left midaxillary line.
   D. fifth intercostal space, left midclavicular line.

FOOD FOR THOUGHT

46. How will you ensure that your patients don't feel awkward or embarrassed when you do ECGs or chest exams?

Copyright © 2025, Elsevier, Inc. All rights reserved.

19 Analysis and Monitoring of Gas Exchange

WORD WIZARD

Match the following quality terms to their definitions.

Definitions	Terms
1. Examining the repeatability of results.	A. Quality control
2. Comparing the values with a known value.	B. Bias
3. Errors of precision.	C. Imprecision
4. Another term associated with errors of precision.	D. Random error
5. A trend or abrupt shift in data outside the limits.	E. Systematic error
6. An oblique or diagonal line.	F. Preanalytical error
7. Problems that occur prior to testing a sample.	G. Precision
8. CLIA standards are an important example.	H. Accuracy

MEET THE OBJECTIVES

Answer the following questions.

9. In your own words, explain how an electrochemical analyzer converts the number of O_2 molecules (PO_2) into a measurable reading.

10. Name the two common types of electrochemical analyzers.

    A. _____

    B. _____

11. Explain the differences between the two types of analyzers in terms of principle of operation and response time.

105

Copyright © 2025, Elsevier, Inc. All rights reserved.

12. Describe the two-step process for calibrating an O_2 analyzer.

13. What is the gold standard of gas exchange analysis? What does this mean?

14. List four reasons that explain why the radial artery is the preferred site for ABG sampling.

A. _____

B. _____

C. _____

D. _____

15. Describe the modified Allen test and give the definition of a positive result.

A. _____

B. _____

16. Name four other sites you can use if the radial artery is unavailable or has a poor pulse.

A. _____

B. _____

C. _____

D. _____

17. How long should you wait after changing the F_iO_2 before performing an ABG on a patient with healthy lungs? On a patient with COPD?

A. _____

B. _____

18. Name the four things you can do to avoid most preanalytical sampling errors.

A. _____

B. _____

C. _____

D. _____

Copyright © 2025, Elsevier, Inc. All rights reserved.

19. What precaution should you take when handling any laboratory specimen?

20. If you wanted to measure actual hemoglobin saturation, what type of analyzer would be needed?

   _____

21. What is the range of accuracy for most commercially available pulse oximeters?

   _____

22. Describe three noninvasive ways you can determine the reliability of a pulse oximeter at the bedside.

   A. _____

   B. _____

   C. _____

23. What action could you take to verify the results when pulse oximetry is unreliable or does not confirm suspicions about the patient's clinical state?

24. What are the two most common errors committed during capillary sampling?

   A. _____

   B. _____

25. Explain what variables are reliable and unreliable in capillary sampling compared to arterial sampling.

26. What are the primary advantages and disadvantages of transcutaneous gas monitoring over arterial sampling?
   A. Advantages

      1. _____

      2. _____

   B. Disadvantages

      1. _____

      2. _____

Copyright © 2025, Elsevier, Inc. All rights reserved.

27. When would you choose a pulse oximeter for monitoring an infant's oxygenation status over a transcutaneous monitor?

28. When would the transcutaneous monitor be preferred over the pulse oximeter?

29. What are the normal values for end-tidal CO_2 for healthy individuals and how do they compare with values for arterial CO_2?

30. An end-tidal CO_2 of "0" may indicate a serious problem. Name two life-threatening causes of a "0" value for end-tidal CO_2.

    A. _____

    B. _____

31. While performing end-tidal CO_2 measurements, you notice that the baseline does not return to "0" on inspiration. Interpret this result.

32. While performing end-tidal CO_2 measurements, you notice that no real plateau is reached. Give two possible interpretations of this result.

    A. _____

    B. _____

SUMMARY CHECKLIST

33. What are the three most common causes of O_2 analyzer malfunctions?

    A. _____

    B. _____

    C. _____

Copyright © 2025, Elsevier, Inc. All rights reserved.

34. Blood gases provide more information than other methods of gas exchange analysis. What are the three general areas that a blood gas helps to assess?

A. _____

B. _____

C. _____

35. What is the maximum ideal time between ABG sampling and analysis?

_____

36. What are the two primary benefits and hazards of indwelling peripheral arterial lines?
    A. Benefits

    1. _____

    2. _____

    B. Hazards

    1. _____

    2. _____

37. What is point-of-care testing, and what are the potential benefits of this method of testing blood samples? Name a potential problem or drawback.

38. What is the difference between capnography and capnometry?

39. Indwelling arterial, central venous, or pulmonary artery catheters are widely used in the ICU. Please list the two main benefits and two main drawbacks of these invasive lines.
    A. Benefits

    B. Drawbacks

Copyright © 2025, Elsevier, Inc. All rights reserved.

Chapter **19** **Analysis and Monitoring of Gas Exchange**

Case 1

A 34-year-old firefighter is brought to the emergency department for treatment of smoke inhalation while fighting a house fire. His heart rate is 126 beats/min, and respirations are 28 breaths/min and labored. SpO_2 is 100% on 6 L/min via nasal cannula. Blood pressure is 145/90 mm Hg. Breath sounds are coarse with inspiratory crackles in both bases. The patient's face is smudged with soot, and he is coughing up sputum with black specks in it.

40. What clinical signs of hypoxemia does the patient display?

41. Explain why the pulse oximeter is reading 100% despite these signs.

42. What is the most probable cause of the hypoxemia?

43. What blood test would you recommend to confirm your suspicions?

Case 2

A premature infant is receiving supplemental O_2. Her physician is concerned about the effects of hyperoxia on her lungs and eyes. The infant is being monitored by a pulse oximeter, which shows a saturation of 100%.

44. What range of PaO_2 is possible with an SpO_2 of 100%?

Copyright © 2025, Elsevier, Inc. All rights reserved.

45. What type of noninvasive monitoring would you recommend in this situation?

Case 3

An elderly patient is admitted for acute exacerbation of his long-standing COPD. He is wearing a nasal cannula with a flow rate of 2 L/min.

46. What is the simplest way to quickly assess his oxygenation status?

47. Why would you recommend arterial blood gas sampling for this patient?

Case 4

A patient was riding his motorcycle without a helmet when he crashed. Now he has a head injury and is being mechanically ventilated. His physician asks you to make recommendations regarding monitoring his gas exchange.

48. What are the advantages of using capnometry to monitor carbon dioxide in this situation?

49. Where would you place the capnometer probe in the ventilator circuit?

Copyright © 2025, Elsevier, Inc. All rights reserved.

50. During monitoring, you notice that the capnograph does not return to "0" when the patient inhales. What does this indicate?

51. A few minutes later, the patient's exhaled CO_2 levels begin to rise. So does his blood pressure. The patient becomes agitated. What action would you take?

52. Why do rising CO_2 levels cause increases in intracranial pressure?

WHAT DOES THE NBRC SAY?

Circle the best answer.

53. A respiratory therapist is preparing to perform pulse oximetry. Which of the following would be *least* beneficial for assessing accuracy of the device?
    A. Checking the capillary refill time
    B. Assessing skin color and temperature
    C. Performing an Allen test on the patient
    D. Assessing pulse rate

54. Which of the following would you perform after obtaining an arterial blood gas sample?
    1. Remove air bubbles from the sample.
    2. Mix the sample by rotating the syringe.
    3. Maintain site pressure for at least 1 minute.
    4. Add heparin to the sample.
        A. 1 only
        B. 1 and 2 only
        C. 1, 2, and 3 only
        D. 1, 2, 3, and 4

55. A pulse oximeter is being used to monitor a patient who was rescued from a fire. The SpO_2 is 90%; however, the patient is unconscious and shows signs of respiratory distress. What additional test should the RT recommend?
    A. CT scan
    B. Electrolyte measurement
    C. Co-oximetry
    D. Hemoglobin and hematocrit levels

Copyright © 2025, Elsevier, Inc. All rights reserved.

56. A polarographic O_2 analyzer fails to calibrate when exposed to 100% O_2. The first action the respiratory therapist should take would be to
    A. replace the battery.
    B. replace the membrane.
    C. replace the fuel cell.
    D. try another O_2 source.

57. An infant is placed on a transcutaneous O_2 monitor. The TcPO$_2$ is reading 40 mm Hg less than the PaO$_2$ obtained from an arterial sample. All of the following could cause this problem *except*
    A. improper calibration of the transcutaneous electrode.
    B. room air contamination of the transcutaneous electrode.
    C. inadequate heating of the skin at the electrode site.
    D. inadequate perfusion of the skin at the electrode site.

58. Which of the following analyzers is calibrated to a value of zero when exposed to room air?
    A. Clark electrode
    B. Galvanic O_2 analyzer
    C. Capnometer
    D. Geisler type of nitrogen analyzer

59. Which of the following would be most useful in assessing proper tube placement following endotracheal intubation?
    A. Transcutaneous monitoring
    B. Arterial blood gas analysis
    C. Pulse oximetry
    D. End-tidal CO_2 monitoring

60. Complications of arterial puncture include all of the following *except*
    A. pulmonary embolus.
    B. hematoma.
    C. infection.
    D. nerve damage.

61. A galvanic O_2 analyzer is being used as a check of the ventilator system to measure the delivered F_iO_2. The set F_iO_2 is 40%; however, the analyzer is reading 32%. Which of the following is the most likely cause of this discrepancy?
    A. The batteries in the analyzer need to be changed.
    B. The electrode membrane has water condensation on its surface.
    C. The analyzer needs to be calibrated.
    D. The ventilator requires servicing.

62. Which of the following will affect the accuracy of pulse oximeter measurements?
    1. Increased bilirubin levels
    2. Decreased hematocrit levels
    3. Dark skin pigmentation
    4. Exposure to sunlight
        A. 1 and 2 only
        B. 2 and 3 only
        C. 3 and 4 only
        D. 2, 3, and 4 only

63. An arterial blood gas sample is drawn from a patient who is breathing room air. Analysis reveals the following results:

pH	7.45
PaCO$_2$	35 mm Hg
PaO$_2$	155 mm Hg

    Which of the following best explains these results?
    A. Too much heparin was added to the sample.
    B. An air bubble has contaminated the sample.
    C. Analysis of the sample was delayed for more than 60 minutes.
    D. The patient was hyperventilating during the puncture.

Copyright © 2025, Elsevier, Inc. All rights reserved.

64. Which of the following sites would be the best for continuous monitoring of exhaled carbon dioxide during mechanical ventilation?
    A. Exhalation valve
    B. Inspiratory side of the ventilator circuit
    C. Expiratory side of the ventilator circuit
    D. Endotracheal tube connector

65. Which of the following is true concerning the use of a transcutaneous PO_2 monitor?
    A. $TcPO_2$ should be checked with arterial blood samples.
    B. The skin temperature control should be maintained at 37°C.
    C. The site should be changed every 24 hours.
    D. The low calibration point is determined using room air.

FOOD FOR THOUGHT

66. How would you modify your technique if you had to perform ABGs on a patient receiving anticoagulants?

67. Why can you use a capnometer during CPR but not a pulse oximeter?

 Copyright © 2025, Elsevier, Inc. All rights reserved.

20 Pulmonary Function Testing

WORD WIZARD

Match the right terms or abbreviations with the correct definition.

Terms/Abbreviations	Definitions
1. DLCO	A. Volume inspired with a normal breath.
	B. Greatest amount of air you can breathe in 12 to 15 seconds.
2. ERV	C. Largest amount of air the lungs can hold.
3. VT	D. Fastest flow rate generated at the very beginning of forced exhalation.
4. IRV	E. Milliliters of gas the lung can transfer to the blood.
5. RV	F. Amount of air you can exhale after a maximum inspiration.
	G. Ratio of volume exhaled in 1 second to total volume exhaled.
6. TLC	H. Average expiratory flow during the early part of forced exhalation.
7. VC	I. Amount of air you can inhale after a normal exhalation.
8. IC	J. Amount of air you can inhale after a normal inspiration.
	K. Air left in the lungs after a maximum exhalation.
9. FRC	L. Air left in the lungs after a normal exhalation.
10. MVV	M. Amount of air you can forcefully exhale after a maximum inspiration
11. FVC	N. Average expiratory flow during the middle part of forced exhalation.
12. PEF	O. Volume of air you can forcefully exhale in 1 second.
13. $FEF_{200\text{-}1200}$	P. Amount of air you can exhale after a normal exhalation.
14. FEV_1	
15. $FEF_{25\%\text{-}75\%}$	
16. FEV_1/FVC	

Copyright © 2025, Elsevier, Inc. All rights reserved.

Put the four lung volumes and four lung capacities into perspective with their normal values in a healthy adult. Use the box provided. MEMORIZE this information! It will serve you well on your board examinations!

A	E	C	B
	F		
	G	D	
	H		H

17. Fill in the names and normal values that go with each letter in the box.

	VOLUME/CAPACITY	VALUE
A.		
B.		
C.		
D.		
E.		
F.		
G.		
H.		

MEET THE OBJECTIVES

Answer these questions to find out if you have grasped the important points for each area of lung testing.

Lung Volumes

18. Which volumes *cannot* be measured with a spirometer?

_____

19. Which capacities *cannot* be measured with a spirometer?

_____

Copyright © 2025, Elsevier, Inc. All rights reserved.

20. Name the three tests used to determine the volumes and capacities that cannot be measured.

A. _____

B. _____

C. _____

21. What is thoracic gas volume?

22. How will volumes or capacities obtained by helium dilution or nitrogen washout differ from those obtained with a body plethysmograph for a patient with air trapping?

23. What effect will an air leak have on the values obtained by helium dilution or nitrogen washout?

Spirometry

24. What four variables are used to calculate normal values for spirometry?

A. _____

B. _____

C. _____

D. _____

25. You must produce acceptable results that provide valid, reliable information based on how long the patient exhales, how closely multiple tests correlate, and how fast the patient starts the maneuver. Fill in the details for each of the criteria below:

A. Duration: _____

B. Variance of two best FVCs: _____

C. Satisfactory start: _____

D. Minimum number: _____

Copyright © 2025, Elsevier, Inc. All rights reserved.

26. Which FVC should you report? Which FEV_1?

    A. FVC: _____

    B. FEV_1: _____

27. Which flow rate is the greatest? _____

28. Which flow rate represents large airways? _____

29. Which flow rate represents the middle range? _____

30. A spirometer is considered accurate if the volume is verified to be within what percentage of a known value?

31. What device is used to verify the volume of a spirometer? _____

32. What is the normal value for MVV? How is this test performed? _____

Diffusion

33. What gas is usually used to measure the lung's ability to transfer gas to the blood?

_____

34. What other special gas is used in this test? Why?

_____

_____

35. What blood test results are needed to ensure accuracy of diffusion studies?

_____

_____

INTERPRETATION FUNDAMENTALS

36. There are two major categories of pulmonary disease. Fill in the chart below to compare the effects of each category.

	CATEGORY	ANATOMY	PHASE	PATHOLOGIC CONDITION	MEASURE
A.	Obstructive				
B.	Restrictive				

37. Fill in the corresponding percentage of predicted values for the degrees of impairment.

Degree of Impairment	% Predicted Value
Normal	_____
Mild	_____
Moderate	_____
Moderately severe	_____
Severe	_____

Copyright © 2025, Elsevier, Inc. All rights reserved.

38. Compare the FEV_1/FVC ratios you would see in normal, obstructed, and restricted patients.

A. Normal: _____

B. Obstructed: _____

C. Restricted: _____

CASE STUDIES

Case 1

Spirometry is performed on a 24-year-old woman who complains of a "tight chest" and cough. Simple spirometry shows the following:

Test	Actual	Predicted	% Predicted
FVC	3.2 L	4 L	80%
FEV_1	1.6 L	3.2 L	50%
FEV_1/FVC	50%	70%	

39. Interpretation? _____

40. What test should be performed in light of the results and the clinical information?

_____

Case 2

A 34-year-old respiratory care student is required by his instructor to undergo pulmonary function testing as part of a course. Here are the results:

Test	Actual	Predicted	% Predicted
FVC	3.9 L	4.8 L	81%
FEV_1	3.1 L	4.1 L	76%
FEV_1/FVC	79%	70%	

41. Interpretation? _____

42. What pulmonary function test would you suggest performing now?

Case 3

A 60-year-old shipyard worker complains of dyspnea on exertion and dry cough. Here are his spirometry results.

Test	Actual	Predicted	% Predicted
FVC	2 L	4 L	50%
FEV_1	1.5 L	3.4 L	44%
FEV_1/FVC	75%	70%	
TLC	2.4	4.8	50%

119

Copyright © 2025, Elsevier, Inc. All rights reserved.

43. Interpretation? _____

44. What additional test would be helpful?

45. What additional history would be helpful?

Case 4

A woman in her physician's office complains of dyspnea on exertion. Spirometry and lung volume results show the following.

Test	Actual	Predicted	% Predicted
FVC	1.5 L	3 L	50%
FEV_1	0.75 L	2.5 L	30%
FEV_1/FVC	50%	70%	
TLC	2.6 L	3.8 L	68%

46. Interpretation? _____

47. What additional history would be helpful?

Case 5

A 70-year-old man with a 100-pack-year smoking history complains of a dry cough and dyspnea on exertion. Results of lung tests show the following.

Test	Actual	Predicted	% Predicted
FVC	2.9 L	4.4 L	65%
FEV_1	1.3 L	3.7 L	35%
FEV_1/FVC	59%	70%	
TLC	6.6 L	5.5	120%
FRC	4.5 L	2.2	
RV	3.7 L	1.1 L	
DLCO	16	25	64%

Copyright © 2025, Elsevier, Inc. All rights reserved.

48. Interpretation? Be complete; what specific type of disease is suggested?

49. What disease state do the lung volumes and history suggest?

_____

50. Why is the vital capacity lower than predicted?

_____

For additional practice, be sure to check out the case studies in Chapter 19 of your textbook!

WHAT DOES THE NBRC SAY?

Circle the best answer.

51. Which of the following tests would be helpful in assessing the effects of cigarette smoking on the smaller airways?
    A. FVC
    B. $FEF_{25\%-75\%}$
    C. FEV_1
    D. $FEF_{200-1200}$

52. A patient's physician asks you to recommend a pulmonary function test to help assess the effects of a possible tumor in the trachea. Which of the following would you recommend?
    A. Spirometry with volume-time curves
    B. Spirometry before and after bronchodilator
    C. Lung volume studies via nitrogen washout
    D. Spirometry with flow-volume loops

53. A pulmonary function technologist tests a spirometer by injecting 3.0 L of air from a large-volume syringe. The spirometer measures 2.9 L. Which of the following is true regarding this situation?
    A. The results are within normal limits.
    B. The spirometer is not ready to use.
    C. The air was injected too slowly.
    D. The BTPS corrections were not made properly.

54. Which of the following values could be incorrectly calculated?

Test	Actual	Predicted	% Predicted
FVC	4.4 L	4.8 L	92%
FEV_1	3.5 L	4.1 L	80%
FEV_1/FVC	80%	70%	
TLC	5.2 L	5.5	
FRC	2 L	2.4	
ERV	1.2 L	1.2 L	
RV	1 L	1.2 L	

A. TLC
B. FVC
C. FRC
D. RV

Copyright © 2025, Elsevier, Inc. All rights reserved.

55. Which of the following pulmonary measurements is usually the smallest?
    A. Inspiratory capacity
    B. Vital capacity
    C. Functional residual capacity
    D. Total lung capacity

56. The following results were obtained from spirometry of an adult female smoker with chronic bronchitis. What is the correct interpretation?

Test	Actual	Predicted	% Predicted
FVC	3.9 L	4.8 L	81%
FEV$_1$	3.1 L	4.1 L	76%
FEV$_1$/FVC	79%	70%	

    A. Results indicate a mild diffusion defect.
    B. Results are within the normal range.
    C. A mixed obstructive/restrictive defect is present.
    D. Results show obstructive lung disease.

57. After a bronchodilator is administered, what percentage increase in forced spirometric volumes or flow rates is the *minimum* indication that reversible airway obstruction is present?
    A. 5%
    B. 10%
    C. 15%
    D. 20%

58. Which of the following can be measured during spirometric testing?
    A. Residual volume
    B. Tidal volume
    C. Total lung capacity
    D. Functional residual capacity

59. An increased total lung capacity combined with a decreased diffusing capacity is strongly indicative of which of the following conditions?
    A. Emphysema
    B. Pneumonia
    C. Pulmonary fibrosis
    D. Pleural effusion

FOOD FOR THOUGHT

We have just scratched the surface of a complex area of testing. Entire textbooks are devoted to pulmonary function testing! Here are a few more questions to fill up the corners of your brain.

60. What effect does smoking have on the results of a diffusion test? Why?

61. What lung volume or capacity is useful in predicting normal values for incentive spirometry?

Copyright © 2025, Elsevier, Inc. All rights reserved.

21 Review of Thoracic Imaging

OVERVIEW

1. Describe the four tissue densities you can see on a chest radiograph.

   A. Air: _____

   _____

   B. Fat: _____

   _____

   C. Tissue: _____

   _____

   D. Bone: _____

   _____

2. Physicians may order, but RTs can recommend; we all work toward a collaborative plan to care for patients. Name three indications for a chest radiograph.

   Outpatient (clinic or office setting)

   A. _____

   B. _____

   C. _____

   Inpatient (ED, ICU, or medical/surgical patient)

   A. _____

   B. _____

   C. _____

3. Explain "lag" in reference to the chest x-ray.

STEP-BY-STEP

4. The two basic ways to shoot a plain chest film are anterior to posterior (AP) and posterior to anterior (PA). You'll want to know which method was used before you continue your evaluation. Explain the differences between AP and PA.

   A. Where does the film go in relationship to the chest, and where is the energy beam (x-ray machine)?

      1. PA

      2. AP

Copyright © 2025, Elsevier, Inc. All rights reserved.

B. What might happen to the heart in an AP film?

C. If PA films are so much better in quality, why do most of our patients have AP chest x-rays?

5. What structures offer clues to help identify whether the patient's position is straight or rotated?

6. What appearance of the vertebral bodies suggests underexposure?

7. What effect does underexposure have on the appearance of lung tissue?

8. The pleura appear at the edge of the chest wall (although the pleura themselves are usually difficult to see). What are the two major pleural abnormalities detected on the chest film?

A. _____

B. _____

ADVANCED CHEST IMAGING

9. CT = _____

What is the advantage over regular radiographs?

What is CT angiography used for?

Copyright © 2025, Elsevier, Inc. All rights reserved.

10. HRCT = _____

Explain the concept of "slices" and what this technique is good for showing.

11. MRI = _____

What type of tissue in the chest is imaged with this technique?

IDENTIFYING ABNORMALITIES

Evaluation of the Pleura

12. What is the costophrenic angle?_____

13. Describe how you recognize the presence of fluid in the pleural space; what does that angle look like?

14. Which view is most sensitive for detecting pleural fluid? How is the patient positioned to obtain this view?

15. When is sonography (ultrasound) indicated in the evaluation of pleural abnormalities?

Copyright © 2025, Elsevier, Inc. All rights reserved.

16. What other imaging procedure may be helpful? _____

_____

17. Air in the pleural space is always abnormal. Name three common causes of this condition.

A. _____

B. _____

C. _____

18. What breathing maneuver will help identify a small pneumothorax on a chest film? _____

_____

19. Tension pneumothorax is immediately life threatening. Name at least two radiographic signs of tension pneumothorax.

A. _____

B. _____

20. What is the treatment for tension pneumothorax? _____

_____

Evaluation of Lung Parenchyma

21. What are the two components of the lung parenchyma?

A. _____

B. _____

22. How will alveolar infiltrates appear on the chest film?

_____

23. What is the difference between the radiographic appearance of pneumonia and pulmonary hemorrhage?

_____

24. What causes airways to become visible, and what is this sign called?

_____

25. Honeycombing, nodules, and volume loss are all radiographic hallmarks of what type of lung disorder?

_____

26. Describe the silhouette sign. Discuss the difference between a right lower lobe and right middle lobe infiltrate as seen on a chest film.

Copyright © 2025, Elsevier, Inc. All rights reserved.

Pathologies

27. List some of the causes of pulmonary edema.

    Vascular

    A. _____

    B. _____

    C. _____

28. Describe Kerley B lines. When do you see them?

29. What are "bat's wings"? _____

Lost Volume

30. List five important indirect signs of volume loss, or atelectasis, seen on the chest radiograph.

    A. _____

    B. _____

    C. _____

    D. _____

    E. _____

31. You can count on the ribs to tell you about lung volumes. Fill in the chart below based on which anterior ribs you would see above the diaphragm depending on the degree of lung inflation.

	LUNG VOLUME	ANTERIOR RIBS
A.	Poor inspiration	
B.	Good effort	
C.	Hyperinflation	

32. Ribs aren't the only way to assess COPD with hyperinflation. List the two primary and three secondary radiographic signs seen in emphysema.

    A. Primary

        1. _____

        2. _____

    B. Secondary

        3. _____

        4. _____

        5. _____

127

Copyright © 2025, Elsevier, Inc. All rights reserved.

33. Compare the sensitivity of the chest radiograph and computed tomography for detection of obstructive airway disease.

Catheters, Lines, and Tubes
Checking placement of tubes and lines is key for RTs.

34. The endotracheal tube is made of soft plastic. How can the chest film be useful in deciding correct tube position after intubation?

35. In an ideally placed endotracheal tube, where is the distal tip in relation to the carina?

_____

36. Where will the endotracheal tube usually end up if it is placed too far into the trachea?

_____

37. What pulmonary complication may be identified on a chest film when a CVP catheter is placed via the subclavian vein?

_____

38. A pulmonary artery catheter (Swan-Ganz) that is seen to extend too far into the lung fields of a chest radiograph may have what unwanted results?

_____

The Mediastinum
39. Where does the mediastinum lie within the chest?

_____

40. What imaging technique is most favored for assessing mediastinal masses?

_____

Copyright © 2025, Elsevier, Inc. All rights reserved.

Case 1

You are asked to perform postural drainage and clapping on a patient with a large right-sided pulmonary infiltrate. Evaluation of the chest radiograph shows a patchy white density with air bronchograms in the right lung. The right border of the heart is visible in the film.

41. Based on your knowledge of the silhouette sign, in what lobe is the infiltrate located?

_____

42. What diagnosis does the presence of air bronchograms suggest?

_____

43. What physical assessments could confirm the information in the chest film?

Case 2

An elderly man presents in the emergency department with acute exacerbation of his long-standing COPD. A decision is made to intubate him. It is difficult to auscultate breath sounds, and chest movement is minimal; however, your impression is that breath sounds are more diminished on the left. A chest radiograph is obtained, which shows the tip of the endotracheal tube 1 cm above the carina. The left lung field is slightly smaller than the right. Both diaphragms appear flat, and you are able to count eight anterior ribs above the diaphragms.

44. Where should the tip of the tube be in relation to the carina?

_____

45. With regard to the endotracheal tube, what action should you take?

_____

46. What is the significance of the flattened diaphragms and number of ribs seen above the diaphragm?

_____

WHAT DOES THE NBRC SAY?

Circle the best answer.

47. A patient has dyspnea and tachycardia following thoracentesis to treat a pleural effusion. Evaluation of this patient should include a(n) _____ .
    A. CT scan
    B. MRI
    C. chest radiograph
    D. bronchoscopy

Copyright © 2025, Elsevier, Inc. All rights reserved.

48. A pneumothorax would appear on a chest radiograph as a _____.
    A. white area near the lung base
    B. white area that obscures the costophrenic angle
    C. dark area without lung markings
    D. dark area with honeycomb markings

49. The medical record of an intubated patient indicates that the morning chest film shows opacification of the lower right lung field with elevated right diaphragm and a shift of the trachea to the right. These findings suggest _____.
    A. left-sided pneumothorax
    B. right-sided pleural effusion
    C. right mainstem intubation
    D. right-sided atelectasis

50. On a chest radiograph, the tip of the endotracheal tube for an adult patient should be _____.
    A. 2 cm above the vocal cords
    B. 5 cm above the carina
    C. at the carina
    D. 2 cm below the carina

51. What specific type of chest radiograph may be useful in evaluating pleural effusion?
    A. Lateral decubitus position
    B. Apical lordotic position
    C. Lateral upright
    D. PA expiratory film

52. A patient with a history of hypertension presents in the ED with headache, slurred speech, and left-sided weakness. What diagnostic imaging procedure would the respiratory therapist recommend to further evaluate this patient according to the ACLS guidelines?
    A. Computed tomography (CT)
    B. Ultrasound
    C. Angiography with contrast
    D. Magnetic resonance imaging (MRI)

53. A patient with a history of pulmonary pathology and cancer presents with a suspicious mediastinal mass on the chest x-ray. What diagnostic imaging procedure would be useful in gathering further information about the mass?
    A. Computed tomography (CT)
    B. Ultrasound
    C. Angiography with contrast
    D. Magnetic resonance imaging (MRI)

54. Ultrasound is useful in the cardiopulmonary setting for
    1. guiding catheter placement.
    2. evaluation of pleural effusion.
    3. evaluation of pneumonia.
    4. diagnosis of myocardial infarction.
       A. 1 and 2 only
       B. 1 and 3 only
       C. 2 and 4 only
       D. 3 and 4 only

55. A respiratory care practitioner is treating a child with respiratory distress in the emergency department. Which type of diagnostic imaging procedure may be useful for differentiating between epiglottitis and croup in children?
    A. AP chest x-ray
    B. Lateral neck x-ray
    C. MRI
    D. Ultrasound

Copyright © 2025, Elsevier, Inc. All rights reserved.

56. The respiratory therapist is checking a patient-ventilator system in the medical intensive care unit when the high-pressure alarm begins to sound. Breath sounds are absent on the left with good tube placement. Blood pressure is 80/50 mm Hg. SpO_2 is 86% and falling. The heart rate is 160 beats/min. There is a hyperresonant percussion note on the left upper chest. The patient has lost consciousness. What action should the respiratory therapist take at this time?
   A. Call for a STAT portable chest x-ray.
   B. Remove the patient from the ventilator and begin manual ventilation.
   C. Remove the endotracheal tube and begin manual ventilation.
   D. Recommend immediate needle decompression of the chest.

FOOD FOR THOUGHT

57. The author states that patient head position is important in assessing the placement of the tip of an endotracheal tube on a radiograph. What happens to the tube if the head moves up (extension) or the chin goes down (flexion)? How far can the tube move?

Copyright © 2025, Elsevier, Inc. All rights reserved.

22 Flexible Bronchoscopy and the Respiratory Therapist

FLEXIBLE BRONCHOSCOPY

1. List five clinical situations where flexible bronchoscopy (FB) would be indicated.

    A. _____

    B. _____

    C. _____

    D. _____

    E. _____

2. List three absolute and relative contraindications for FB.
   Absolute contraindications

    A. _____

    B. _____

    C. _____

   Relative contraindications

    A. _____

    B. _____

    C. _____

3. What is the goal of sedation during FB?

4. Describe the Mallampati classification.

Copyright © 2025, Elsevier, Inc. All rights reserved.

5. List three vital sign measurements the respiratory therapist should monitor while a patient is sedated for an FB. What else should be monitored?

A. _____

B. _____

C. _____

DIAGNOSTIC BRONCHOSCOPY

6. What is a BAL and when is it indicated?

A. BAL: _____

B. Indication: _____

7. What is the difference between a BAL and bronchial washings?

THERAPEUTIC BRONCHOSCOPY

8. When is rigid bronchoscopy (RB) indicated?

THERMAL ABLATION OF THE ENDOBRONCHIAL LESION

9. Describe the following thermal ablation techniques.

A. Electrocautery: _____

B. Argon plasma coagulation: _____

C. Laser photocoagulation: _____

10. What are the above techniques used for?

Copyright © 2025, Elsevier, Inc. All rights reserved.

11. What should a respiratory therapist consider regarding oxygen delivery during thermal ablation?

12. What are endobronchial stents used for?

13. Describe the two different types of endobronchial stents.

   A. _____

   B. _____

14. List two indications for a self-expanding metallic stent.

   A. _____

   B. _____

BRONCHOSCOPIC INTERVENTIONS

15. What patient population may benefit from bronchial thermoplasty (BT)?

CASE STUDY

You are the respiratory therapist (RT) in the intensive care unit (ICU) of a large urban trauma center. You are about to assist the physician with an FB procedure on an intubated patient who is receiving mechanical ventilation.

16. What preprocedure responsibilities are the RT accountable for to ensure patient safety?

Copyright © 2025, Elsevier, Inc. All rights reserved.

17. What vital signs would you be evaluating during the procedure? Is there anything else the respiratory therapist may assist with during the procedure?

18. What serious complications are possible following this type of procedure?

Circle the best answer.

19. You are preparing a patient for her flexible bronchoscopy procedure. Her weight is 50 kg. What is the total dose of lidocaine that should not be exceeded to help avoid methemoglobinemia?
    A. 300 mg
    B. 350 mg
    C. 400 mg
    D. 450 mg

20. What effects could be seen during a flexible bronchoscopy procedure on an intubated patient receiving mechanical ventilation?
    A. High peak inspiratory pressures
    B. Increase in tidal volume delivery
    C. Acute hypocapnia
    D. High minute ventilation alarm

FOOD FOR THOUGHT

As the field of respiratory therapy advances, the RT will be called on to assist in more complex respiratory procedures. Many procedures directly affect the respiratory system and should be within our area of expertise. This means you need to be constantly studying and always willing to learn new and exciting things. Remember, you need to be the lung expert!

Copyright © 2025, Elsevier, Inc. All rights reserved.

23 Nutrition Assessment

Terms	Definitions
1. _____ Anergy	A. Excess nitrogenous waste in the blood.
2. _____ Anthropometrics	B. Relationship of weight to height.
3. _____ Azotemia	C. So thin that ribs stick out in persistent malnutrition.
4. _____ Basal metabolic rate	D. Energy measurement based on O_2 consumption and CO_2 production.
5. _____ Body mass index	E. Impaired immune response.
6. _____ Indirect calorimetry	F. Body measurements; the most frequently used are height and weight.
7. _____ Cachexic	G. Hourly resting energy consumption after fasting.

MEET THE OBJECTIVES

8. Describe the "most helpful" technique for nutrition assessment dietitians perform in the acute care setting.

9. What does BMI stand for, and what two variables are used to calculate it?

   A. BMI = _____

   B. Variable 1: _____

   C. Variable 2: _____

10. State the range of normal for BMI. (What is *your* BMI? What about your loved ones?)

   _____

Copyright © 2025, Elsevier, Inc. All rights reserved.

11. State the formula for calculating ideal body weight.

    A. Males: _____

    B. Females: _____

    C. Calculate your own ideal body weight:

BIOCHEMICAL INDICATORS

12. Describe why serum proteins are useful as biochemical indicators when assessing nutritional status.

13. Why is monitoring albumin of limited use in assessing effectiveness of nutrition in the critical care setting?

14. What is the most used biomarker for inflammation? What causes this biomarker to increase?

MACRONUTRIENTS

15. Name the three macronutrients that supply the body's energy requirements. State the kilocalories per gram for each.

	MACRONUTRIENT	KILOCALORIES PER GRAM
A.		
B.		
C.		

Copyright © 2025, Elsevier, Inc. All rights reserved.

16. What percentage of patients with acute respiratory failure suffers from malnutrition?

_____

17. List two reasons malnourished patients are difficult to wean from the ventilator.

A. _____

B. _____

18. Why are COPD patients often malnourished?

19. What are the consequences of malnutrition for respiratory muscles and response to hypoxia and hypercapnia?

INDIRECT CALORIMETRY

20. List three conditions where indirect calorimetry may be indicated.

A. _____

B. _____

C. _____

21. What are the contraindications to indirect calorimetry in mechanically ventilated patients?

22. According to the AARC Clinical Practice Guidelines, closed-circuit calorimeters may reduce alveolar volume or increase work of breathing. Explain how these two hazards occur.

Copyright © 2025, Elsevier, Inc. All rights reserved.

23. What actions should be taken to prepare a patient for indirect calorimetry?

    A. 4 hours before the test: _____

    B. 2 hours before the test: _____

    C. 1 hour before the test: _____

24. Describe the most significant problem in performing indirect calorimetry on mechanically ventilated patients.

25. Interpret the following RQs and identify the general nutritional strategy.

	VALUE	INTERPRETATION	GENERAL NUTRITION STRATEGY
A.	> 1		
B.	0.9 to 1		
C.	0.8 to 0.9		
D.	0.7 to 0.8		

26. State the formula for calculating REE using a pulmonary artery catheter. _____

_____

27. What factors are used to adjust predicted REEs in patients? Give one example. (Go to Table 21-5.)

RESPIRATORY CONSEQUENCES

28. COPD patients have special dietary problems. Identify four factors that lead to poor intake in these patients.

    A. _____

    B. _____

    C. _____

    D. _____

29. What is the effect of high-carbohydrate loads on COPD patients?

_____

Copyright © 2025, Elsevier, Inc. All rights reserved.

30. What do the terms "enteral" and "parenteral" mean?

    A. Enteral: _____

    B. Parenteral: _____

31. How would the respiratory therapist confirm suspected aspiration of tube feedings? How is this complication avoided?

    A. Confirmation: _____

    B. Prevention: _____

    _____

    _____

32. Explain what happens when patients receive too much of the following substrates. Give a pulmonary example, please.

    A. Protein: _____

    B. Carbohydrates: _____

    C. Fat: _____

Pulmonary Pathologies

33. In general, COPD patients eat to optimize nutrition.

    A. How often? _____

    B. Calories? _____

34. People with asthma may greatly benefit from what specific type of fatty acids? _____

35. In addition to a lot of calories, what supplements do CF patients need? _____

SUMMARY CHECKLIST

Complete the following sentences by writing in the correct information in the spaces provided.

36. What equation can be used to estimate daily resting energy expenditure?

37. Define malnutrition.

38. For patients with pulmonary disease, what can foods high in carbohydrates cause?

Copyright © 2025, Elsevier, Inc. All rights reserved.

39. Whenever possible, what route should be used for supplying nutrients?

40. How can the likelihood of aspiration during tube feedings can be minimized?

CASE STUDY

A thin, undernourished COPD patient tells you that he has difficulty eating because he gets tired and short of breath during meals. Besides, food just doesn't taste as good now.

41. What eating pattern should be emphasized to this patient?

_____

_____

42. Make some suggestions that would increase his nutrient intake.

_____

_____

43. What other big problem might interfere with the patient's appetite?

_____

_____

WHAT DOES THE NBRC SAY?

44. A respiratory therapist is caring for a 66-year-old male patient with acute exacerbation of COPD. The therapist notes the patient is extremely thin, with ribs obviously showing on his chest. What term should the therapist use to document the patient's appearance?
    A. Malnourished
    B. Cyanotic
    C. Cachexic
    D. Wasted

45. Cystic fibrosis patients may need what dietary supplement to be able to absorb nutrients?
    A. Calcium
    B. Amino acids
    C. Enzymes
    D. Vitamin C

Copyright © 2025, Elsevier, Inc. All rights reserved.

46. What type of nutritional strategy may help in weaning COPD patients from the ventilator?

47. What is the key to indirect calorimetry? What can invalidate the results of the test?

 Copyright © 2025, Elsevier, Inc. All rights reserved.

24 Pneumonia

WORD WIZARD

Write out the definition for each acronym.

CAP _____

NVHAP _____

HAP _____

VAP _____

VAE _____

OK, now put the correct descriptive acronym next to these statements:

This patient got sick at home. _____

This patient got sick while receiving mechanical ventilation. _____

This patient got sick in the hospital. _____

CLASSIFICATION AND PATHOGENESIS

1. Explain the term *contiguous spread*.

2. The textbook definition of nosocomial pneumonia is now subdivided into HAP and VAP. Please describe these new terms *in depth* using the textbook criteria, because they are critical to your understanding of this life-threatening illness.

    A. HAP

    B. VAP

Copyright © 2025, Elsevier, Inc. All rights reserved.

3. What is the most common reason a for a patient developing pneumonia?

4. List two ways nosocomial infections can be prevented.

   A. _____

   B. _____

5. What major mechanism contributed to CAP viral infections?

6. State the two novel strategies mentioned in the book to reduce HAP or VAP in ventilated patients.

   A. _____

   B. _____

7. Give an example of reactivation of a latent infection.

MICROBIOLOGY

8. Why is it so important to know which organisms are commonly associated with pneumonia?

9. Which organism is most commonly identified as the cause of community-acquired pneumonia?

Copyright © 2025, Elsevier, Inc. All rights reserved.

10. List the three most common atypical pathogens.

   A. _____

   B. _____

   C. _____

11. What is considered an appropriate duration for treatment of HAP?

CLINICAL MANIFESTATIONS

12. In addition to fever, list the three respiratory symptoms patients with pneumonia typically exhibit.

   A. _____

   B. _____

   C. _____

13. Describe radiograph abnormalities associated with pneumonia. Why is the chest film of limited use in diagnosing pneumonia in critically ill patients?

RISK FACTORS

14. A number of factors predispose hospital patients to pneumonia, such as poor host defenses from underlying illness. List two

   A. _____

   B. _____

DIAGNOSTIC STUDIES

15. What do the initials BAL stand for? Describe BAL.

   A. BAL = _____

   B. Description: _____

   _____

   _____

145

Copyright © 2025, Elsevier, Inc. All rights reserved.

16. What is the primary medical treatment for pneumonia?

17. When is remdesivir used?

PREVENTION

18. Immunization is one of the primary strategies for preventing community-acquired pneumonia. Individuals are immunized against which organisms?

   A. _____

   B. _____

   C. _____

19. Identify two groups that should receive the pneumococcal vaccine.

   A. _____

   B. _____

20. What positioning technique is useful in preventing pneumonia in patients?

CASE STUDIES

Case 1

A 55-year-old man arrives at the emergency department complaining of chills, fever, and chest pain on inspiration. He is coughing up rusty-colored sputum. He admits to a history of heavy smoking and regular use of alcoholic beverages. Physical examination reveals a heart rate of 125 beats/min, respiratory rate of 30 breaths/min, and temperature of 104°F. He has inspiratory crackles in the right lower lobe. Blood gases reveal a pH of 7.34, $PaCO_2$ of 50 mm Hg, and PaO_2 of 58 mm Hg.

21. What is the most likely diagnosis? Support your answer based on the clinical signs and symptoms.

Copyright © 2025, Elsevier, Inc. All rights reserved.

22. What immediate treatment should you initiate?

23. A patient is seen in the ED with fever, chills, and tachypnea. He states he feels weak and short of breath. The vitals are T 101.4°F, f 28, HR 121, BP 140/96, and SpO$_2$ 88% on room air. What should the respiratory therapist do first?
    A. Obtain a sputum specimen.
    B. Request a chest x-ray.
    C. Place the patient on antibiotics.
    D. Place the patient on oxygen.

24. A 14-year-old is admitted to the medical floor with "acute exacerbation of asthma secondary to lung infection." While administering bronchodilator therapy, the respiratory therapist observes the patient producing moderate amounts of thick yellow phlegm. What should the therapist recommend at this point?
    A. Obtain a sputum specimen.
    B. Request a chest x-ray.
    C. Place the patient on antibiotics.
    D. Place the patient on oxygen.

25. Which of the following mechanisms is the most common cause for bacterial pneumonia?
    A. Inhalation
    B. Aspiration
    C. Contiguous spread
    D. Hematogenous dissemination

26. A person with AIDS presents in the ED with profound hypoxemia, shortness of breath, and nonproductive cough. Physical examination findings suggest bilateral lower lobe pneumonia. Which of the following organisms is most likely to be seen in this particular individual?
    1. *Pneumocystis jiroveci*
    2. *Streptococcus pneumoniae*
    3. *Mycobacterium tuberculosis*
       A. 1 only
       B. 2 and 3 only
       C. 1 and 3 only
       D. 1, 2, and 3

27. New onset of fever accompanied by purulent secretions and a new infiltrate on the chest film in an intubated patient are strongly suggestive of
    A. VAP.
    B. HAP.
    C. CAP.
    D. MDR.

Copyright © 2025, Elsevier, Inc. All rights reserved.

28. The respiratory therapist suspects that one of her ventilator patients is at high risk for developing pneumonia. What general action should the therapist take?
   A. Request a chest x-ray.
   B. Elevate the head of the bed.
   C. Implement the VAP protocol.
   D. Implement an in-line suction catheter.

FOOD FOR THOUGHT

29. What is the role of the RT in educating at-risk populations about methods to prevent pneumonia?

Copyright © 2025, Elsevier, Inc. All rights reserved.

25 Obstructive Lung Disease: Chronic Obstructive Pulmonary Disease (COPD), Asthma, and Related Diseases

CHRONIC OBSTRUCTIVE PULMONARY DISEASE

1. *Chronic obstructive pulmonary disease* is defined by the American Thoracic Society (ATS) by four key concepts. Please elaborate on the following.

   A. Limitation: _____

   B. Progressive: _____

   C. Inflammatory: _____

   D. Systemic: _____

2. According to the National Health Interview Survey data, what percentage of the U.S. population has COPD?

3. How does COPD rank as a leading cause of death in the United States, and why is this condition strikingly different from heart disease or stroke?

Risk Factors and Pathophysiology

4. It is estimated 80% to 90% of cigarette smokers get COPD. What is the other major cause of emphysema?

   _____

5. Briefly explain the protease-antiprotease hypothesis of emphysema.

Copyright © 2025, Elsevier, Inc. All rights reserved.

6. Describe three mechanisms of airflow obstruction in COPD.

A. _____

B. _____

C. _____

Clinical Signs

7. List four common symptoms of COPD.

A. _____

B. _____

C. _____

D. _____

8. Compare the onset of dyspnea in typical cases of COPD with that of α_1-antitrypsin deficiency.

9. What physical change in the chest wall occurs as a result of prolonged hyperinflation?_____

_____

10. List three other late signs of COPD.

A. _____

B. _____

C. _____

11. Compare chronic bronchitis, emphysema, and α_1-antitrypsin deficiency in terms of the following features.

FEATURES	CHRONIC BRONCHITIS	EMPHYSEMA	SEVERE α_1-ANTITRYPSIN DEFICIENCY
Symptoms and Signs			
Chronic cough, phlegm			
Dyspnea on exertion			
Cor pulmonale			
Age of patient at symptom onset			
Family history of COPD			
History of cigarette smoking			

Copyright © 2025, Elsevier, Inc. All rights reserved.

FEATURES	CHRONIC BRONCHITIS	EMPHYSEMA	SEVERE α_1-ANTITRYPSIN DEFICIENCY
Physiologic Function			
Airflow (FEV_1, FEV_1/FVC)			
Lung volumes, residual volume			
Gas exchange, diffusion PaO_2			
$PaCO_2$			
Diffusion capacity			
Static lung compliance			
Chest radiograph			

Management

12. Why would it be important to differentiate asthma from other forms of COPD? List some distinguishing characteristics of each.

    A. Why differentiate?

    B. Features characteristic of COPD:

    C. Features characteristic of asthma:

13. Reversible airflow obstruction is defined as an increase of what amount?

Copyright © 2025, Elsevier, Inc. All rights reserved.

14. Why is bronchodilator therapy recommended for COPD? What types of drugs are used?

A. Why? _____

B. Types of drugs? _____

15. Discuss the role of inhaled steroids (ICS) in COPD. Are there any concerns with inhaled corticosteroid use?

16. List the important elements of managing an acute exacerbation of COPD due to purulent bronchitis.

17. Fill in the chart regarding the severity of COPD is graded based on the degree of airflow obstruction.

Stage	Description
I	
II	
III	
IV	

18. What is the primary goal of pulmonary rehabilitation? _____

_____

19. A comprehensive smoking cessation program usually includes what three elements?

A. _____

B. _____

C. _____

Copyright © 2025, Elsevier, Inc. All rights reserved.

20. Three treatments for COPD have been shown to prolong survival. Please elaborate.
    A. Oxygen:

    B. Quitting smoking:

    C. Lung volume reduction surgery (LVRS):

21. What is the relationship between bronchodilator therapy and home oxygen therapy?

22. You need to know the indications for continuous oxygen. Please give the correct values for
    A. Resting PaO$_2$: _____
    B. Hematocrit: _____
    C. ECG: _____

ASTHMA

Overview

23. Define asthma.

Copyright © 2025, Elsevier, Inc. All rights reserved.

24. What percentage of people in the United States is believed to have asthma?

Etiology and Pathogenesis

25. Airway inflammation and bronchial hyperreactivity result in airflow obstruction. What are some triggers?

_____

_____

_____

26. What happens when a patient with asthma inhales an allergen to which he or she is sensitized?

27. Describe early and late asthmatic reactions (EAR and LAR, respectively).
    A. EAR:

    B. LAR:

Copyright © 2025, Elsevier, Inc. All rights reserved.

28. What factor plays a key role in suggesting and establishing a diagnosis of asthma?_____

_____

29. List four classic symptoms of asthma.

    A. _____

    B. _____

    C. _____

    D. _____

30. List five conditions that can mimic the wheezing of asthma.

    A. _____

    B. _____

    C. _____

    D. _____

    E. _____

31. Bronchial provocation is the specialized test used to demonstrate obstruction in patients with suspected asthma who are symptom-free at the time of testing. Name the drug used for this test and what response indicates hyperresponsiveness.

    A. Drug: _____

    B. Response: _____

Management

32. Explain control of asthma in terms of the following criteria:

    A. Symptoms: _____

    _____

    B. β_2-agonists: _____

    _____

    C. Exercise: _____

    _____

    D. PEFR/FEV$_1$: _____

    _____

    E. Exacerbations: _____

    _____

33. Give the criteria and actions for green, yellow, and red peak flow zones.

	ZONE	PEFR % PREDICTED	TREATMENT/ACTION
A.	Green		
B.	Yellow		
C.	Red		

Copyright © 2025, Elsevier, Inc. All rights reserved.

34. Compare the use of inhaled corticosteroids and bronchodilators in treating asthma.

35. Name the two common side effects of inhaled steroids and two ways to control them.

   A. _____

   B. _____

   C. Control/reduce side effects:

      1. _____

      2. _____

36. Leukotriene modifiers such as montelukast sodium (Singulair) are popular and useful for which categories of asthma? Do these drugs replace steroids?

   _____

37. What type of drug is the first-line treatment for all types of acute bronchospasm? _____

   _____

38. Using anticholinergics such as ipratropium may be helpful in management of what type of asthma?

39. List three factors you should monitor in a patient hospitalized with acute asthma.

   A. _____

   B. _____

   C. _____

40. Management of asthma should be aggressive, including two specific types of medications along with oxygen. Discuss the use of β-agonists and steroids in this specific situation.

   A. β-agonists: _____

   _____

   B. Steroids: _____

   _____

Copyright © 2025, Elsevier, Inc. All rights reserved.

41. How can you prevent allergic reactions in patients with asthma through immunotherapy?

42. What is exercise-induced asthma (EIA)? List two prophylactic drug treatments.

  A. EIA = _____

  B. Prophylaxis: _____

    1. _____

    2. _____

43. Define occupational asthma. What is the most common cause?

44. What is the only way to eliminate occupational asthma once an individual is sensitized?

  _____

45. What drug is particularly helpful in the treatment of cough-variant asthma?

  _____

46. List three medications that may be helpful in treating nocturnal asthma.

  A. _____

  B. _____

  C. _____

47. What recommendations would you make to a patient who has aspirin sensitivity?

Copyright © 2025, Elsevier, Inc. All rights reserved.

48. What is the effect of pregnancy on women with asthma?

49. Discuss the use of asthma medications during pregnancy.

50. GER (most of us call it GERD) can also play a role in asthma. Any ideas on how to help?

51. A surprising number of people with asthma have nose and sinus problems. What types of inhalers do they need?

BRONCHIECTASIS

52. What is the clinical hallmark of bronchiectasis?

_____

53. What test is now considered definitive for diagnosing bronchiectasis?

_____

54. List the three major anatomic patterns seen in bronchiectasis.

A. _____

B. _____

C. _____

Copyright © 2025, Elsevier, Inc. All rights reserved.

55. List the two primary treatments for bronchiectasis.

A. _____

B. _____

And if these don't work, the patient needs to have _____

CASE STUDIES

Case 1

A 70-year-old man's chief complaint is dyspnea on exertion. He has a smoking history of two packs per day for the past 50 years. He has a barrel-shaped chest and significantly decreased breath sounds. His chest radiograph shows hyperinflation, especially in the apices, flattened diaphragms, and a small heart. He admits to a morning cough but denies significant sputum production.

56. What is the most likely diagnosis?

_____

57. Calculate the patient's pack-years. _____

58. What factor should you focus on to help the patient control his condition?

_____

Case 2

A 60-year-old man has smoked a pack of cigarettes per day since he was a teenager. He complains of a chronic productive cough that is producing thick, yellow sputum. He is admitted to the medical floor with a fever and shortness of breath. Blood gases reveal pH of 7.35, $PaCO_2$ of 50 mm Hg, and PaO_2 of 57 mm Hg. Physical examination shows pedal edema, distended neck veins, and use of accessory muscles of ventilation. He has scattered wheezing and rhonchi on auscultation.

59. What type of COPD is most likely in this case?

_____

60. What should you do with his sputum the next time he coughs productively?

61. What is the immediate respiratory treatment in this case?

Copyright © 2025, Elsevier, Inc. All rights reserved.

62. What respiratory medications would you recommend?

Case 3

A 44-year-old man complains of dyspnea on exertion. He is a nonsmoker but drinks wine with his meals. He has a barrel-shaped chest and very decreased breath sounds. His chest radiograph shows hyperinflation, especially in the bases. History reveals that his father and uncle both died of "lung problems."

63. What is the most likely cause of the patient's COPD symptoms? Justify your answer based on the information presented.

64. What treatments are available for this condition?

Case 4

A 15-year-old boy complains that he cannot catch his breath when he exercises. He states that he coughs a lot, especially in the winter. His breath sounds are clear, and his physical examination is unremarkable.

65. What do you suspect is the problem? _____

_____

66. How could a definitive diagnosis be made?

Copyright © 2025, Elsevier, Inc. All rights reserved.

Use the following data to answer questions 67 through 72.

A 20-year-old woman who has a history of asthma is brought to the emergency department in respiratory distress. Your assessment of the patient reveals the following:

pH	7.47
$PaCO_2$	33 mm Hg
PaO_2	72 mm Hg
HCO_3^-	23 mEq/L
RR	28
HR	115
PEFR	200 L/min

67. Which of the following breath sounds would you expect to hear in this patient?
    A. Inspiratory crackles
    B. Expiratory wheezing
    C. Inspiratory stridor
    D. Expiratory rhonchi

68. The arterial blood gas results indicate the presence of
    A. acute respiratory alkalosis.
    B. acute metabolic alkalosis.
    C. chronic respiratory acidosis.
    D. acute respiratory acidosis.

69. You are asked to initiate oxygen therapy. What would you recommend?
    A. Simple mask at 10 L/min
    B. Nonrebreathing mask at 15 L/min
    C. Nasal cannula at 2 L/min
    D. Air-entrainment mask at 0.50 F_IO_2

70. What therapy would you recommend after the oxygen is in place?
    A. 2 puffs ipratropium (Atrovent) via MDI
    B. 2.5 mg albuterol (Proventil) via SVN
    C. Intravenous theophylline administration
    D. Intravenous antibiotics

71. Blood gases are repeated 30 minutes after the oxygen therapy is initiated.

pH	7.42
$PaCO_2$	38 mm Hg
PaO_2	86 mm Hg
HCO_3^-	23 mEq/L
RR	24
HR	88
PEFR	210 L/min

    Which of the following has shown significant improvement based on this information?
    A. Compliance
    B. Resistance
    C. Oxygenation
    D. Ventilation

72. Intravenous steroids and repeated bronchodilators have been given. The patient is now receiving F_IO_2 of 0.40.

pH	7.34
$PaCO_2$	53 mm Hg
PaO_2	74 mm Hg
HCO_3^-	26 mEq/L
RR	18
HR	125
PEFR	110 L/min

Copyright © 2025, Elsevier, Inc. All rights reserved.

What would you suggest at this point?
A. Increase F_iO_2 to 0.50
B. Continuous nebulization of bronchodilators
C. Administration of intravenous bicarbonate
D. Intubation and mechanical ventilation

73. A patient with COPD and CO_2 retention is admitted for an acute exacerbation of her disease. The physician requests your suggestion for initiating oxygen therapy. Which of the following would you recommend?
A. Nasal cannula at 6 L/min
B. Air-entrainment mask at 28%
C. Simple mask at 2 L/min
D. Partial rebreathing mask at 8 L/min

74. A PFT on a 65-year-old woman indicates airflow obstruction with mild air-trapping. The patient is coughing up thick sputum. Which of the following diagnoses is most likely?
A. Cystic fibrosis
B. Pneumonia
C. Pulmonary fibrosis
D. Bronchiectasis

75. A PFT on a 56-year-old man with a history of smoking shows increased TLC and RV. The Dlco is reduced. What diagnosis is suggested by these findings?
A. Emphysema
B. Pneumonia
C. Sarcoidosis
D. Pneumoconiosis

76. Spirometry is performed before and after bronchodilator administration. Which of the following indicates a therapeutic response?
1. FEV_1 increased by 10%.
2. FVC increased by 300 ml.
3. PEFR increased by 5%.
   A. 1 only
   B. 2 only
   C. 1 and 2 only
   D. 1 and 3 only

FOOD FOR THOUGHT

77. Because only 15% of smokers show big declines in airflow, why should we encourage all patients to quit smoking?

78. What is omalizumab (Xolair), and how does it work for asthma?

Copyright © 2025, Elsevier, Inc. All rights reserved.

26 Interstitial Lung Disease

WORD WIZARD

WORD WIZARD

Match the correct definition with the correct term.

Terms	Definitions
_____ 1. Asbestosis	A. Formation of scar tissue in the lung without known cause
_____ 2. Corticosteroids	B. Respiratory disorder characterized by fibrotic infiltrates in the lower lobes
_____ 3. Drug-related lung disease	C. Inflammatory reaction provoked by inhalation of organic dusts
_____ 4. Lymphangioleiomyomatosis	D. Lung disease caused by chemotherapy agents, for example
_____ 5. Hypersensitivity pneumonitis	E. Asbestosis, chronic silicosis, and coal workers' pneumoconiosis
_____ 6. Idiopathic pulmonary fibrosis	F. Restrictive disorder associated with pleural abnormalities and lung tumors
_____ 7. Interstitial lung disease	G. Disorder of unknown origin that results in formation of epithelioid tubercles
_____ 8. Interstitium	H. Hormones associated with control of body processes
_____ 9. Occupational ILD	I. A rare disorder of abnormal smooth muscle tissue proliferating around small airways leading to severe obstruction and destruction of alveoli with resultant thin-walled cyst formation
_____ 10. Organizing pneumonitis	J. The area between the capillaries and the alveolar space
_____ 11. Pulmonary Langerhans cell histiocytosis	K. The revised term for *bronchiolitis obliterans organizing pneumonia*
_____ 12. Sarcoidosis	L. Disorder caused by long-term exposure to sand and stone dust
_____ 13. Silicosis	M. Nodules are star-shaped and destroy adjacent lung tissue

CLINICAL SIGNS AND SYMPTOMS OF ILD

14. Patients with interstitial lung disease (ILD) of many different etiologies will usually present with which two common complaints?

    A. _____

    B. _____

15. Describe the breath sounds typically heard in ILD. _____

    _____

Copyright © 2025, Elsevier, Inc. All rights reserved.

16. List the late signs of ILD.

_____

17. Physical signs of underlying connective tissue disease include what three features?

A. _____

B. _____

C. _____

18. Describe the classic and late radiographic findings in idiopathic pulmonary fibrosis. What are the late-stage findings?

A. Classic: _____

B. Late: _____

19. Discuss the effects of ILD on the following pulmonary function variables.

	VARIABLE	EFFECT OF ILD
A.	FEV_1	
B.	FVC	
C.	FEV_1/FVC	
D.	DLCO	
E.	Lung volumes	
F.	Compliance	

SPECIFIC TYPES OF ILD

20. List the three most common types of occupational ILD.

A. _____

B. _____

C. _____

21. What do these examples have in common?

22. Why is pulmonary involvement in connective tissue disorders often undetected until late in the course of the disease?

Copyright © 2025, Elsevier, Inc. All rights reserved.

23. List three common connective disorders associated with lung disease.

A. _____

B. _____

C. _____

24. What is the name for chronic exposure to inhaled organic material that results in progressive scarring of the lung?

_____

25. What factor is critical to identifying the cause of this condition?

_____

26. What is meant by the term "idiopathic"? _____

_____

27. Let's compare the two idiopathic lung diseases discussed in the text.

		Idiopathic Pulmonary Fibrosis (IPF)	Sarcoidosis
A.	Age		
B.	Symptoms		
C.	Treatment		
D.	Prognosis		

28. Discuss the common areas of treatment for hypersensitivity pneumonitis and occupational lung disease.

29. What is the primary drug therapy for ILD? _____

_____

30. What is the most common respiratory therapy modality for ILD? _____

_____

31. What is the only therapy shown to prolong life in end-stage ILD? _____

_____

Copyright © 2025, Elsevier, Inc. All rights reserved.

Case 1

A 48-year-old man is admitted for dyspnea on exertion and a dry cough of unknown origin. The chest radiograph shows bilateral reticulonodular infiltrates. Pulse oximetry indicates mild hypoxemia on room air. History reveals that the patient is a hay farmer.

32. What is the most likely diagnosis?

_____

33. What is the most likely cause of the lung disease? What are some other possible causes?

Case 2

A retired Pearl Harbor shipyard worker states that he has had a cough for some time but recently began expectorating some blood. He has bibasilar inspiratory crackles, with otherwise clear breath sounds. A chest radiograph shows reticulonodular infiltrates in both lower lobes. The radiologist also notes the presence of a small right-sided pleural effusion and the presence of pleural plaques and pleural fibrosis. PFTs reveal a normal FEV_1 %, decreased TLC and RV, and a decreased D_{LCO}.

34. What is the most likely pulmonary diagnosis?

_____

35. What other information would be helpful in making a determination?

36. What type of disorder is suggested by the PFT results?

Copyright © 2025, Elsevier, Inc. All rights reserved.

37. A patient with a history of sarcoidosis presents in the emergency department with shortness of breath.
    Vital signs are T 99, P 114, f 32, BP 138/88, and SpO_2 82%. The respiratory care practitioner would
    A. administer oxygen via nasal cannula at 2 L/min.
    B. request a STAT portable AP chest x-ray.
    C. perform a STAT ABG.
    D. administer albuterol.

FOOD FOR THOUGHT

38. What is the general term for all lung diseases that cause a reduction in lung volumes without a reduction in flow

    rates? _____

Copyright © 2025, Elsevier, Inc. All rights reserved.

27 Pleural Diseases

WORD WIZARD

Chapter 27 introduces lots of important new terms. Match these pleural puzzlers to their definitions.

Terms	Definitions
1. _____ Bronchopleural fistula	A. Pleural effusion high in protein
2. _____ Chylothorax	B. Air leak from the lung to the pleural space
3. _____ Empyema	C. Membrane covering the surface of the chest wall
4. _____ Exudative effusion	D. Pleural fluid rich with triglycerides from a ruptured thoracic duct
5. _____ Hemothorax	E. Pleural pain
6. _____ Parietal pleura	F. Pus-filled pleural effusion
7. _____ Pleural effusion	G. Blood in the pleural space
8. _____ Pleurisy	H. Abnormal collection of fluid in the pleural space
9. _____ Pleurodesis	I. Pneumothorax without underlying lung disease
10. _____ Pneumothorax	J. Air under pressure in the pleural space
11. _____ Primary spontaneous pneumothorax	K. Procedure that fuses the pleura to prevent pneumothorax
12. _____ Reexpansion pulmonary edema	L. Air in the pleural space
13. _____ Secondary spontaneous pneumothorax	M. Occurs when the lung is rapidly inflated after compression by pleural fluid
14. _____ Tension pneumothorax	N. Pneumothorax that occurs with underlying lung disease
15. _____ Thoracentesis	O. Low-protein effusion caused by CHF or cirrhosis
16. _____ Transudative pleural effusion	P. Chest wall puncture for diagnostic or therapeutic purposes
17. _____ Visceral pleura	Q. Membrane that lines the lung surface

THE PLEURAL SPACE

18. Which nerves supply the costal pleura? Which nerves supply the diaphragmatic pleura?

Copyright © 2025, Elsevier, Inc. All rights reserved.

19. Describe both the visceral and parietal pleura. Where do the two meet and become a single, continuous pleural membrane?

20. Are normal intrapleural pressure positive or negative, and what effect does this have on fluid movement?

21. Explain why pleural pressures are different at the apex and lung bases.

PLEURAL EFFUSIONS

22. Give a brief explanation of how each of the following conditions can cause transudative pleural effusions.
    A. CHF:

    B. Hypoalbuminemia:

Copyright © 2025, Elsevier, Inc. All rights reserved.

C. Liver disease:

D. Lymph obstruction:

E. CVP line:

23. What is the most common cause of clinical pleural effusions?

    _____

24. What is the general cause of exudative pleural effusions?

    _____

25. Give a brief explanation of the cause of these exudative pleural effusions.

    A. Parapneumonic

    B. Malignant

Copyright © 2025, Elsevier, Inc. All rights reserved.

C. Chylothorax

D. Hemothorax

26. What change in pulmonary function is associated with pleural effusion?

_____

27. In what specific portion of the upright chest film is pleural effusion visualized?

_____

28. Describe the specific type of chest film used to improve visualization of pleural effusions.

29. What type of imaging is the most sensitive test for identification of pleural effusions?

_____

30. List the three major risks of thoracentesis.

A. _____

B. _____

C. _____

31. Identify the purpose of each of the chambers in the three-bottle chest tube drainage system shown on the next page.

A. _____

B. _____

C. _____

Copyright © 2025, Elsevier, Inc. All rights reserved.

To wall suction-
60 cm H₂O

−20 cm H₂O

−20 cm H₂O

To pleural
space

Chest tube
−20 cm H₂O

cm H₂O

20

10

The standard three-bottle system is the basis for all commercial chest tube drainage systems.

PNEUMOTHORAX

32. List two symptoms that are common to almost all cases of pneumothorax.

    A. _____

    B. _____

33. What is the most common type of traumatic pneumothorax, and how is it treated? Give three examples.

34. Compare blunt and penetrating chest trauma as cause of pneumothorax. How does treatment differ in these two situations?

35. What special technique may be helpful to visualize pneumothorax in a newborn?

    _____

36. Compare the two major types of spontaneous pneumothorax.

Copyright © 2025, Elsevier, Inc. All rights reserved.

37. Tension pneumothorax can be a life-threatening medical emergency. It is a common board exam item. Please give short clear explanations for items A through D.

A. Definition

B. Radiographic finding

C. Clinical signs

D. Treatment

38. How does oxygen administration assist in resolution of a pneumothorax?

39. What is BPF? How does mechanical ventilation perpetuate this problem? What special modes of ventilation may be indicated?

A. BPF = _____

B. Ventilators perpetuate BPF by: _____

C. Adjust ventilator for BPF patient by: _____

Copyright © 2025, Elsevier, Inc. All rights reserved.

A mathematics instructor with a history of CHF is admitted with a complaint of pain on inspiration. Her respirations are rapid and shallow, and her heart rate is 104 beats/min. The pulse oximeter shows a saturation of 93% on room air. Breath sounds are very decreased on the right side, with crackles in the left base. Chest wall movement is markedly less on the right. The chest radiograph shows opacification of the right lung, with shift of mediastinal structures to the left. Diagnostic percussion reveals a dull note on the right side.

40. What do you think is wrong with this patient's right lung? Support your conclusion with at least five pieces of information from the case.

    A. I think the patient has a _____ because

        1. _____

        2. _____

        3. _____

        4. _____

        5. _____

41. What would you recommend as the first respiratory intervention?

    _____

42. How could this disorder be resolved?

Copyright © 2025, Elsevier, Inc. All rights reserved.

A tall, thin young male respiratory care instructor is admitted with a complaint of pain on inspiration. His respirations are rapid and shallow, and his heart rate is 104 beats/min. The pulse oximeter shows a saturation of 93% on room air. Breath sounds are very decreased on the right side, and clear in the left base. Chest wall movement is markedly less on the right. The chest radiograph shows a dark area without lung markings on the right side, with a shift of mediastinal structures to the left. Diagnostic percussion reveals increased resonance on the right side.

43. What do you think is wrong with this patient's right lung? Support your conclusion with at least five pieces of information from the case.

    A. I think this patient has a _____ because

        1. _____

        2. _____

        3. _____

        4. _____

        5. _____

44. What would you recommend as the first respiratory intervention?

45. How could this disorder be resolved?

WHAT DOES THE NBRC SAY?

Circle the best answer.

46. Immediately after insertion of a central line via the subclavian vein, an intubated patient becomes dyspneic. The respiratory therapist should recommend which of the following diagnostic tests?
    A. 12-lead ECG
    B. Chest radiograph
    C. ABG
    D. Bedside spirometry

Copyright © 2025, Elsevier, Inc. All rights reserved.

47. The middle bottle of a three-bottle chest drainage system is used for which of the following?
   A. Water seal
   B. Fluid collection
   C. Means of applying vacuum to the chest
   D. Measurement of improvement of the pneumothorax

48. A chest tube is placed anteriorly between the second and third ribs. The tube is probably intended to treat a
   A. chylothorax.
   B. hemothorax.
   C. transudative pleural effusion.
   D. pneumothorax.

49. A patient is suspected of having a pleural effusion. Which x-ray position is most appropriate to confirm this diagnosis?
   A. AP chest film
   B. Lateral decubitus chest film
   C. Apical lordotic chest film
   D. PA chest film

50. Thoracentesis is performed and 1500 ml of fluid is removed from the right chest. Which of the following is likely to occur as a result?
   A. Pulmonary edema in the right lung
   B. Stridor and respiratory distress
   C. Pneumothorax in the right lung
   D. Atelectasis in the right lung

51. All of the following would be useful in differentiating right mainstem intubation from left-sided pneumothorax *except*
   A. chest radiograph.
   B. diagnostic percussion.
   C. auscultation.
   D. lung compliance measurement.

52. Following an IPPB treatment, a COPD patient complains of sudden severe chest pain. What is the respiratory therapist's first priority in this situation?
   A. Notify the physician of the problem.
   B. Initiate oxygen therapy.
   C. Recommend a chest radiograph.
   D. Perform an arterial blood gas.

53. A patient develops subcutaneous emphysema following a motor vehicle accident involving multiple rib fractures. What action should the respiratory therapist take in this situation?
   A. Perform bedside spirometry.
   B. Initiate oxygen therapy.
   C. Recommend a chest radiograph.
   D. Perform an arterial blood gas.

FOOD FOR THOUGHT

54. What is meant by the term "ascites"? Besides causing effusions, how could ascites affect respiratory function?

55. What is subcutaneous emphysema, and what relationship does it have to pneumothorax?

Copyright © 2025, Elsevier, Inc. All rights reserved.

28 Pulmonary Vascular Disease

1. How many people develop thromboembolic disease each year in the United States? _____

2. Where do most of pulmonary embolisms (PE) arise from?

3. Explain how PE affects the heart and lungs as they try to function together. (Just give the basic idea.)

4. What is the primary hemodynamic consequence of PE?

5. List the two most common symptoms of PE.

   A. _____

   B. _____

   C. _____

6. List the three most frequent physical findings associated with PE.

   A. _____

   B. _____

   C. _____

7. List the two most common ECG abnormalities associated with PE.

   A. _____

   B. _____

Copyright © 2025, Elsevier, Inc. All rights reserved.

8. How is the chest radiograph helpful in diagnosing pulmonary embolism?

9. How helpful are arterial blood gases (ABGs) in ruling out PE? What benefit does an ABG provide in these cases?

10. One rapid blood test has been developed to help rule out embolism. Why isn't D-dimer as good for some in-patients?

11. Which test is considered the "gold standard" for the diagnosis of DVT?

_____

FINDING PE

12. Because of the high mortality rate, it is important to make a definitive diagnosis of pulmonary embolus. What test is reliable in confirming this diagnosis?

_____

13. What is the relationship of the ventilation ($\dot{V}$) and perfusion ($\dot{Q}$) portions of scans in making a high-probability diagnosis of PE?

ASSESS AND TEST

14. Prophylaxis for DVT is either pharmacologic or mechanical. Give three examples of each.
    A. Pharmacologic prophylaxis

    1. _____

    2. _____

    3. _____

 Copyright © 2025, Elsevier, Inc. All rights reserved.

B. Mechanical prophylaxis

    1. _____

    2. _____

    3. _____

15. What is the standard pharmacologic therapy for existing DVT or PE? What is the mechanism of action? What are the risks?

    A. Drug:

    _____

    B. Action:

    _____

    C. Risks:

    _____

16. How are thrombolytics different from anticoagulants? Can they be given together?

17. Give three examples of thrombolytic drugs.

    A. _____

    B. _____

    C. _____

18. List the mechanical options available for treatment of massive PE.

19. When are vena cava filters indicated?

Copyright © 2025, Elsevier, Inc. All rights reserved.

20. Define pulmonary hypertension (PH).

21. Describe the epidemiology of idiopathic pulmonary hypertension in terms of age, gender, symptoms, mortality, and genetic factors.

    A. Age: _____

    B. Gender: _____

    C. Symptoms: _____

    D. Most common causes: _____

22. How is PH diagnosed?

23. Why is it so important to provide oxygen as needed to keep up the patient's saturations in this condition?

24. Which drug treatment is given via inhalation? _____

25. Explain the role of alveolar hypoxia in the development of pulmonary hypertension.

26. What other factors seen in COPD contribute to this condition? _____

Copyright © 2025, Elsevier, Inc. All rights reserved.

27. What is the only treatment that improves survival in patients with COPD and pulmonary hypertension? What treatments might help?

CASE STUDY

A 60-year-old man underwent total knee replacement. Two days after surgery, he complains of dyspnea and anxiety. Physical examination reveals a heart rate of 110, respiratory rate of 28, blood pressure of 115/80 mm Hg, and SpO_2 of 93% on room air. Breath sounds are clear except for faint inspiratory crackles in both bases.

28. Why is this patient at risk for PE?

29. What additional diagnostic tests would be helpful in ruling out other potential pulmonary problems?

30. What treatment would you provide as a respiratory therapist?

_____

31. What medical treatment should be initiated if a diagnosis of PE is confirmed?

_____

WHAT DOES THE NBRC SAY?

Circle the best answer.

32. A patient who is being mechanically ventilated shows an increased V_D/V_T ratio. Which of the following disorders could be responsible?
    A. Atelectasis
    B. Pneumonia
    C. Pulmonary embolism
    D. Pleural effusion

33. Which of the following is the most appropriate test to confirm the presence of a suspected PE?
    A. Chest radiograph
    B. $\dot{V}/\dot{Q}$ scan
    C. Bronchogram
    D. Arterial blood gas

Copyright © 2025, Elsevier, Inc. All rights reserved.

34. A ventilation/perfusion scan reveals a defect in perfusion in the right lower lobe without a corresponding decrease in ventilation. Which of the following is the most probable diagnosis?
    A. Right lower lobe atelectasis
    B. Acute pulmonary embolus
    C. Pneumothorax
    D. Pneumonia

FOOD FOR THOUGHT

35. Discuss the *Westermark sign* and the *Hampton hump* in the confirmation of PE.

Copyright © 2025, Elsevier, Inc. All rights reserved.

29 Acute Respiratory Distress Syndrome (ARDS)

WORD WIZARD

Write out the definitions of terminology found in Chapter 29.

1. ALI: _____

2. APRV: _____

3. ARDS: _____

4. CHF: _____

5. ECMO: _____

6. $ECCO_2R$: _____

7. TRALI: _____

8. HFV: _____

9. MODS: _____

10. PEEP: _____

11. VILI: _____

MEET THE OBJECTIVES

General Considerations

12. For each of the following general categories, name two common conditions leading to hydrostatic pulmonary edema:

	CATEGORY	CONDITIONS
A.	Cardiac	1. 2.
B.	Vascular	1. 2.
C.	Volume Overload	1. 2.

Copyright © 2025, Elsevier, Inc. All rights reserved.

13. List four primary and four secondary risk factors or "triggers" for ARDS.
   A. Primary (direct injury)
      1. _____
      2. _____
      3. _____
      4. _____

   B. Secondary (indirect injury)
      1. _____
      2. _____
      3. _____
      4. _____

14. Compare the recommended definitions for ARDS using the AECC criteria and the Berlin criteria.

	AECC Criteria (1994)	Berlin Criteria (2012)
Timing of onset		
Risk factor		
Exclusion of hydrostatic edema		
Hypoxemia		
Chest imaging		

15. What five areas should be addressed to prevent further lung injury in ARDS?
   A. _____
   B. _____
   C. _____
   D. _____
   E. _____

Ventilator Strategies

16. How does optimal PEEP differ from PEEP that delivers the best PaO_2?

17. We can attempt to avoid barotrauma by maintaining plateau pressures below what value?

   _____

18. PEEP should be adjusted to maintain what F_iO_2 and PaO_2?

   _____

184

Copyright © 2025, Elsevier, Inc. All rights reserved.

19. What is the tidal volume range used in ARDS patients?

_____

20. What is meant by "permissive hypercapnia"? What is the goal of this ventilator strategy?

21. In what condition is permissive hypercapnia contraindicated? Why?

_____

_____

Innovative Strategies

22. A man is 6 feet tall. He has ARDS. What is the formula? The PBW? The right volume?
    A. Formula:

    B. Calculate the PBW.

    C. What range of tidal volume do you have to work with according to ARDSNet?

23. What mode of mechanical ventilation is best for patients with ARDS to prevent against lung damage?

24. How can patient positioning be radically altered to improve gas exchange?

25. Both ECMO and $ECCO_2R$ facilitate gas exchange via what type of device?

_____

26. Exogenous surfactant is helpful in treating infant respiratory distress syndrome and when surfactant is washed out of the adult lung. What's the story on using this with ARDS in adults?

185

Copyright © 2025, Elsevier, Inc. All rights reserved.

Pharmacologic Treatments

27. Surfactant is not currently recommended for ARDS. What patient group does respond to surfactant administration?

_____

28. What was the potential role of nitric oxide (NO) in treating ARDS?

29. What is the consequence of sudden discontinuation of inhaled NO?

_____

CASE STUDIES

Case 1

A 5-foot, 6-inch, 143-lb (65-kg) teenager had a cut on his lower leg. Now he is in the ICU with a temperature of 103°F, blood pressure of 80/50 mm Hg, heart rate of 120 beats/min, and SpO_2 of 88% on 100% oxygen. His pulmonary capillary wedge pressure is 14 mm Hg, and cardiac output is 8 L/min. Breath sounds reveal coarse crackles throughout the lungs, and his bronchoalveolar lavage fluid contains a very high protein level. The patient is intubated and currently is being ventilated with a tidal volume of 800 ml, frequency of 14, and PEEP of 0.

30. What is the most likely diagnosis? Why?

_____

31. With regard to the oxygenation status, what changes would you recommend?

_____

32. With regard to the volume, what changes would you recommend?

_____

WHAT DOES THE NBRC SAY?

Circle the best answer.

33. Which of the following would be useful in treating an elevated shunt in a patient with ARDS who is being mechanically ventilated?
    A. Initiating IMV mode
    B. Optimizing PEEP
    C. Increasing the F_iO_2
    D. Adding expiratory retard

34. Which of the following indicates the optimal PEEP setting?

	PEEP	PaO_2	Cardiac Output
A.	5 cm H_2O	53 mm Hg	4.5 L/min
B.	10 cm H_2O	60 mm Hg	4.3 L/min
C.	15 cm H_2O	74 mm Hg	3.8 L/min
D.	20 cm H_2O	88 mm Hg	3.4 L/min

Copyright © 2025, Elsevier, Inc. All rights reserved.

35. A patient is admitted to the ICU with a diagnosis of pulmonary edema. Which of the following breath sounds is consistent with this diagnosis?
    A. Inspiratory stridor
    B. Inspiratory crackles
    C. Expiratory rhonchi
    D. Pleural friction rub

36. A patient with ARDS is being ventilated with the following settings:

Mode	Assist Control
F_iO_2	0.80
Frequency	10
PEEP	5 cm H_2O
V_t	500 ml
SpO_2	82%

Which of the following would you recommend as possible ways to improve oxygenation?
    A. Increase the tidal volume.
    B. Increase the PEEP.
    C. Increase the F_iO_2.
    D. Increase the rate.

37. Which of the following would provide necessary information regarding fluid management in a critically ill patient with cardiogenic pulmonary edema?
    A. Bedside pulmonary function testing
    B. Intake and output measurements
    C. Daily weights
    D. Pulmonary artery catheter

38. Chest radiograph changes associated with noncardiogenic pulmonary edema include: _____
    1. pleural effusion.
    2. bilateral infiltrates.
    3. enlarged left ventricle.
        A. 1 and 2 only
        B. 2 only
        C. 2 and 3 only
        D. 1 and 3 only

FOOD FOR THOUGHT

39. Lower inflection point (LIP or P_{flex}) is useful in setting appropriate PEEP and tidal volume levels. What is meant by the term LIP? How is it determined?

_____

187

Copyright © 2025, Elsevier, Inc. All rights reserved.

30 Respiratory Management of Trauma, Obesity, Near Drowning, and Burns

WORD WIZARD

Match the correct definition with the correct term.

Terms	Definitions
_____ 1. Penetrating trauma	A. Laryngospasm with closure of the glottis prevents aspiration of large amounts of fluid in the lungs.
_____ 2. Blunt trauma	B. Occurs with sudden immersion in water cooler than 25°C.
_____ 3. Morbid obesity	C. Scale used to assess traumatic brain injury.
_____ 4. Obesity hypoventilation syndrome	D. Multifocal fractures of one or more ribs.
_____ 5. Dry drowning	E. BMI greater than 45 kg/m².
_____ 6. Wet drowning	F. High force applied to a small surface area of the body, such as with a gunshot.
_____ 7. Glasgow Coma Scale	G. Occurs when laryngospasm lessens with unconsciousness, leading to the aspiration of fluid.
_____ 8. Tension pneumothorax	H. Affects the most severely obese patients who acquire a reduced chemosensitivity, impairing their ventilatory response to hypoxemia and hypercapnia.
_____ 9. Flail chest	I. Develops when the pleural lesion acts as a one-way valve allowing the entrance of air into the pleural space and progressively trapping air in the expanding pleural cavity.
_____ 10. Cold shock cardiac-respiratory reflexes	J. High force applied over a larger body surface, such as the case of a head-on motor vehicle accident

LIFE-THREATENING TRAUMA

11. How many yearly hospital admissions in the United States are the result of trauma?

12. What are the three categories of the Glasgow Coma Scale?

A. _____

B. _____

C. _____

188

Copyright © 2025, Elsevier, Inc. All rights reserved.

13. If blunt force trauma is suspected, what intervention should the RT and the medical team perform immediately?

14. You are the RT working in the emergency department of a Level-1 trauma center when a patient presents with blunt trauma to the thoracic region. What are you worried about?

15. What therapeutic approach would you take to manage the patient in Question #14?

OBESITY

16. Fill in the chart below categorizing the Body Mass Index of an individual.

BMI category	Range
Normal BMI	
Obesity	
Severe obesity	
Morbid obesity	
Super obesity	

Copyright © 2025, Elsevier, Inc. All rights reserved.

17. List four diseases associated with obesity.

A. _____

B. _____

C. _____

D. _____

18. What is one of the most challenging aspects of ventilatory management of obese patients?

NEAR DROWNING

19. How many drowning deaths occurred in the United States between 2010 and 2019? In adults, what was the general cause?

20. Explain the cold shock cardiac reflexes.

21. What effects does the inhalation of fresh water have on the respiratory system?

22. What effects does the inhalation of salt water have on the respiratory system?

Copyright © 2025, Elsevier, Inc. All rights reserved.

BURNS

23. What three categories does the respiratory assessment of a burn patient include?

    A. _____

    B. _____

    C. _____

24. How effective is a pulse oximeter in measuring arterial oxygen saturation in an inhalation injury?

CASE STUDY

Bastian is a 26-year-old male patient who was involved in a motor vehicle crash. He was not wearing a seat belt and sustained significant chest trauma as well as a broken tibia. He has been stabilized and is in the intensive care unit. He is currently unable to get out of bed.

25. What respiratory complications is Bastian at risk of developing?

26. Bastian's nurse reports to you that he is having trouble clearing his secretions. What is a likely cause for his difficulty?

27. During rounds the next day the attending physician asks for your respiratory treatment plan for Bastian. What interventions would you discuss with the attending physician?

SUMMARY CHECKLIST

28. What interventions do any clinical signs of upper airway injury from smoke inhalation generally require?

Copyright © 2025, Elsevier, Inc. All rights reserved.

29. What syndrome should all obese patients be assessed for in addition to sleep apnea?

30. Generally, gas exchange abnormalities in near drowning are a result of fluid shifts and the activation of what type of mediators?

31. Your patient was just intubated following a house fire that resulted in an inhalation injury. What should you set the F_iO_2 at when the patient is placed on mechanical ventilation?
    A. 0.5
    B. 0.6
    C. 0.8
    D. 1.0

32. A patient was intubated and mechanically ventilated following a stab wound to the chest. Suddenly, the high-pressure alarm is triggered and simultaneously the patient's heart rate increases and blood pressure drops. What is the likely cause?
    A. Inappropriately set alarms on the ventilator
    B. A hemopneumothorax has developed
    C. Acute bronchospasm
    D. Pleural effusion

33. Most adult drownings are a result of
    A. diving injury.
    B. alcohol.
    C. inability to swim.
    D. swift water currents.

34. Which of the following should a respiratory therapist use to assess the severity of possible carbon monoxide poisoning?
    A. Complete blood count
    B. Pulse oximetry
    C. Hemoximetry
    D. Peak expiratory flow rates

35. A 42-year-old female has been pulled from a house fire and has arrived in the ED. She has burns on her face and chest with edema of the oropharynx and audible stridor. Her blood gas reveals respiratory alkalosis with moderate hypoxemia. Which of the following should the respiratory therapist recommend?
    A. Initiate 2.5 mg of albuterol via nebulizer.
    B. Administer 2.25% racemic epinephrine via nebulizer for the stridor.
    C. Intubate the patient.
    D. Apply oxygen via nasal cannula at 4 L/min.

FOOD FOR THOUGHT

36. Why is early tracheostomy often advocated in burn patients with suspected inhalation injuries?

Copyright © 2025, Elsevier, Inc. All rights reserved.

31 Acute Heart Failure

WORD WIZARD

Write out each of these acronyms.

1. ACE: _____

2. ACS: _____

3. AHF: _____

4. ARB: _____

5. LV – AHF: _____

6. MAPSE: _____

7. HFpEF: _____

8. STEMI: _____

9. TAPSE: _____

PATHOPHYSIOLOGY OF ACUTE HEART FAILURE

10. What is the main clinical manifestation of left ventricular heart failure?

11. What are the two predominant mechanisms of organ dysfunction in patients with acute heart failure?

12. Compare and list the main symptoms of LV – AHF with RV – AHF.

Copyright © 2025, Elsevier, Inc. All rights reserved.

13. How does the body attempt to compensate for the hypoperfusion caused by a decrease in cardiac output? What are the subsequent affects of this compensation of oxygen consumption?

14. What is the goal of acute heart failure treatment?

15. List three things that can be determined when measuring cardiac output in the patient with AHF.

A. _____

B. _____

C. _____

16. What imaging study is typically performed when active cardiac ischemia is suspected?

CASE STUDY

Case 1

A 65-year-old, 143-lb (65-kg) woman was intubated after presenting in the emergency department with pulmonary edema, severe respiratory distress, and AHF. Now she is in the ICU with a temperature of 97°F, blood pressure of 80/50 mm Hg, heart rate of 120 beats/min, and an SpO_2 of 90% on 60% oxygen. Her pulmonary capillary wedge pressure is 24 mm Hg and cardiac output is 3 L/min. Breath sounds reveal coarse crackles throughout the lungs. The patient is intubated and currently being ventilated with a tidal volume of 500 ml, frequency of 14, and PEEP of 10 cmH$_2$O.

17. What is the most likely diagnosis? What's the underlying cause?

_____

18. With regard to the oxygenation status, what changes would you recommend?

Copyright © 2025, Elsevier, Inc. All rights reserved.

19. CHF-associated pulmonary edema is due to elevated _____ pressures in the

pulmonary _____.

20. ARDS-associated pulmonary edema results from _____ injury
to the lungs.

WHAT DOES THE NBRC SAY?

21. A patient is complaining of shortness of breath with bilateral course lung sounds in the bases, a chest radiograph
shows diffuse alveolar infiltrates, and lung echocardiography reveals multiple B-lines. The following data is
available:
CVP: 13 mmHg
PCWP: 24 mmHg

A respiratory therapist should recommend administering
A. Albuterol
B. Nitric oxide
C. Diuretics
D. A fluid bolus

22. A patient with congestive heart failure tells the respiratory therapist that she feels like she can breathe better at night
when she sleeps sitting in her chair. This is most indicative of what breathing pattern?
A. Kussmaul
B. Hyperpnea
C. Cheyne-Stokes respiration
D. Orthopnea

23. Monitoring serum electrolytes is indicated in patients who are receiving which of the following medications?
A. Diuretics
B. Surfactants
C. Beta blockers
D. ACE inhibitors

FOOD FOR THOUGHT

24. What is the main mechanism demonstrated to produce respiratory failure during AHF?

25. If the reduction in left ventricle compliance as a consequence of either left ventricular wall stiffening or ventricular
compression is not the mechanism causing an increase in pulmonary artery occlusion pressure, what is another possible cause?

26. What is a non-pharmacologic intervention for patients with acute heart failure when medical therapy failed to stabi-
lize or recover the patient?

Copyright © 2025, Elsevier, Inc. All rights reserved.

32 Lung Cancer

Match each of the following abbreviations with their definition.

1.	MRI	A. Staging system based on the size of the tumor, the presence and position of abnormal lymph nodes, and the presence or absence of metastasis
2.	CT	B. Radiographic techniques that produce a film that represents a detailed cross-section of tissue structure.
3.	TNM	C. Imaging technique using magnetic disturbance of tissue to obtain images.
4.	PET	D. Computerized radiographic technique that uses radioactive substances to examine the metabolic activity of various body structures.

MEET THE OBJECTIVES

5. How many cases of lung cancer were newly diagnosed in the United States in 2022? How many cases does the WHO estimate occur worldwide each year?

    A. _____

    B. _____

6. What percentage of cancer deaths are caused by smoking tobacco?

7. Compare lung cancer deaths of men and women in the United States.

8. Compare high school senior daily cigarette smoking rates compared to e-cigarette use.

Copyright © 2025, Elsevier, Inc. All rights reserved.

9. What is another name for passive exposure to smoke?

_____

10. Describe the health risks of passive exposure to smoke.

11. Besides smoking, list four other major influences linked to an increase in lung cancer.

    A. _____

    B. _____

    C. _____

    D. _____

12. What is meant by the term *apoptosis?*

13. List the four major histopathologic types of lung cancer along with the epidemiology they represent and a brief description of the cells.

TYPE OF CANCER	EPIDEMIOLOGY	DESCRIPTION
A. Adenocarcinoma		
B. Squamous cell		
C. Small cell		

CLINICAL FEATURES

14. List the four common sites of metastasis of cancer originating in the lungs.

    A. _____

    B. _____

    C. _____

    D. _____

15. What percentage of patients with lung cancer are asymptomatic at the time of presentation?

_____

16. Local tumor growth in the central airways may cause many symptoms. Name four that a respiratory therapist can easily recognize.

    A. _____

    B. _____

    C. _____

    D. _____

197

Copyright © 2025, Elsevier, Inc. All rights reserved.

17. Patients with pleural or chest wall involvement will typically have what two symptoms?

    A. _____

    B. _____

18. Explain "Pancoast syndrome."

19. Give three examples of paraneoplastic syndromes commonly associated with lung cancers. Describe briefly, please.

    A.

    B.

    C.

DIAGNOSIS

20. Two methods are used to obtain tissue for confirmation. Please describe both of the following.

    A. Flexible bronchoscopy (FB):

    B. Transthoracic needle biopsy (TNB):

Copyright © 2025, Elsevier, Inc. All rights reserved.

21. Why is tumor staging so important?

22. How is small cell cancer staged?

23. What's the consensus on mass screenings for people at high risk for lung cancer?

TREATMENT

24. Why is surgical resection the treatment of choice for all non–small-cell lung cancers?

_____

25. What patients are *not* candidates for surgery in terms of staging?

_____

26. How are respiratory therapists involved in determining candidates for surgery?

_____

27. What test values for percent predicted postoperative (PPO) and Dlco suggest a patient may (or may not!) safely undergo lobectomy or pneumonectomy?

28. Name the two nonsurgical therapy modalities.

   A. _____

   B. _____

199

Copyright © 2025, Elsevier, Inc. All rights reserved.

29. What is meant by *palliative* therapy? Give examples.

   A. Medications:

   B. Radiotherapy:

   C. Bronchoscopy:

ROLE OF THE RESPIRATORY THERAPIST

Respiratory therapists don't perform surgery or administer chemotherapy or radiation to cancer patients. Still, many of these patients have preexisting lung disease or have airway problems.

30. Describe the role RTs play in

   A. Nicotine intervention:

   B. Diagnosis:

   C. Support:

Copyright © 2025, Elsevier, Inc. All rights reserved.

SUMMARY CHECKLIST

Complete the following sentences by writing the correct information in the spaces provided.

31. What is the leading cause of cancer deaths in the United States?

32. What is the addictive chemical in tobacco?

33. What is the most effective way to prevent lung cancer?

CASE STUDIES

Chapter 32 has excellent case studies in the form of Mini-Clinis. Four of these cases are particularly useful to the respiratory therapist.

Pancoast's Tumor

34. Will you be caring for patients with weakness and drooping eyelids? How is care different?

Paraneoplastic Syndrome

35. Confusion and generalized weakness are signs of what type of serious neurologic vascular accident?

Evaluating Surgical Risk

36. What therapy modalities might improve lung function prior to surgery for lung resection?

Copyright © 2025, Elsevier, Inc. All rights reserved.

37. What methods of diagnosis might be useful for the patient with copious amounts of clear, frothy sputum?

FOOD FOR THOUGHT

38. Besides lung cancer, what are the other significant health risks of smoking?

Copyright © 2025, Elsevier, Inc. All rights reserved.

33 Neuromuscular and Other Diseases of the Chest Wall

WORD WIZARD

WORD WIZARD

Try matching these diseases to their definitions.

Diseases	Definitions
_____ 1. Ankylosing spondylitis	A. Neuromuscular conduction disorder that particularly affects the face, throat, and respiratory muscles.
_____ 2. Amyotrophic lateral sclerosis	B. Chronic inflammatory disease that fuses the spine and affected joints.
_____ 3. Flail chest	C. Muscle-wasting disease characterized by delayed relaxation of contracted groups.
_____ 4. Guillain-Barre syndrome	D. Degenerative disease of motor neurons characterized by progressive atrophy.
_____ 5. Lambert-Eaton syndrome	E. Inflammation of muscles caused by a rheumatologic disorder.
_____ 6. Myasthenia gravis	F. Unstable chest, as a result of rib fractures, that exhibits paradoxical movement on inspiration.
_____ 7. Myotonic dystrophy	G. Idiopathic polyneuritis characterized by ascending weakness.
_____ 8. Polymyositis	H. Abnormal curvature of the spine that may compromise ventilation.
_____ 9. Kyphoscoliosis	I. Neuromuscular conduction disorder associated with underlying malignancy.

MEET THE OBJECTIVES

10. Neuromuscular abnormalities affect four major groups of muscles that may result in respiratory problems. List these four groups.

   A. _____

   B. _____

   C. _____

   D. _____

11. List the three common complaints of patients with respiratory muscle weakness as a result of neuromuscular disease.

   A. _____

   B. _____

   C. _____

Copyright © 2025, Elsevier, Inc. All rights reserved.

12. Pulmonary function testing of patients with neuromuscular disease and otherwise normal lung tissue will demonstrate what type of ventilatory defect?

_____

13. What three specific tests are most useful in monitoring ventilatory function in patients with neuromuscular weakness?

A. Assess volumes with _____

B. Assess muscle strength via _____

C. Assess hypoxemia and hypercapnia with _____

14. What signs and symptoms suggest performing nocturnal oximetry or formal sleep testing?

_____

15. What is the primary treatment for severe respiratory muscle weakness? What is diaphragmatic pacing?

A. Primary treatment: _____

B. Diaphragmatic pacing: _____

Specific Neuromuscular Diseases

16. What is myopathic disease? Give two examples of common myopathies.

A. What is it? _____

B. Example 1 _____

C. Example 2 _____

17. What general category of drugs is used to treat myasthenia gravis?

_____

18. What surgical treatment may be effective in some cases of myasthenia gravis?

_____

19. List four predisposing factors to Guillain-Barré syndrome (GBS).

A. _____

B. _____

C. _____

D. _____

20. Bilateral interruption of the phrenic nerves that results in diaphragmatic paralysis is seen in what type of injury?

_____

21. Reversible unilateral diaphragmatic paralysis occurs frequently following what commonly performed surgery?

_____

Copyright © 2025, Elsevier, Inc. All rights reserved.

22. Describe the chest radiographic presentation of unilateral diaphragmatic paralysis.

23. Define the high and middle/low classification of cervical cord lesions.

   A. High:

   _____

   B. Middle/low:

   _____

24. Describe the muscle groups affected by each of the following spine injuries.

Level	Muscle Groups
A. C1-2	_____
B. C3-5	_____
C. C4-8	_____
D. T1-12	_____
E. T7-L1	_____

25. What type of breathing is the hallmark sign of significant diaphragmatic weakness?

   _____

26. What are the two basic types of strokes?

   A. _____

   B. _____

27. Give examples of the effect on the respiratory system of strokes in the following locations in the brain.

Location	Effect on Respiration
A. Cerebral cortex	_____
B. Bilateral hemispheric infarct	_____
C. Lateral medulla	_____
D. Mid pons	_____

28. Aside from problems similar to stroke, brain trauma can cause what respiratory "fluid" problems?

   A. _____

   B. _____

Copyright © 2025, Elsevier, Inc. All rights reserved.

29. Describe these two chest wall deformations that often occur together.

   A. Kyphosis:

   B. Scoliosis:

30. Describe the ventilatory defects and pulmonary function changes associated with severe kyphoscoliosis.

   A. Ventilation:

   B. Pulmonary function:

31. Describe the paradoxical chest motion that is the hallmark of flail chest.

32. Name three other pulmonary injuries frequently associated with flail chest.

   A. _____

   B. _____

   C. _____

  Copyright © 2025, Elsevier, Inc. All rights reserved.

33. Regardless of the physiologic mechanisms behind respiratory dysfunction, what are the mainstays of treatment for flail chest?

A. _____

B. _____

C. _____

SUMMARY CHECKLIST

Write the correct response in the spaces provided.

34. What are respiratory dysfunctions in many neuromuscular diseases?

35. List two signs and symptoms of muscle weakness.

_____

_____

36. Give an example of what PFTs typically seen in patients with neuromuscular disease would show.

37. Fill in the chart below regarding the comparison of Myasthenia Gravis and Guillain-Barré Syndrome.

	MG	GBS
Pattern of muscle involvement		
Triggers		
Timeline of weakness		
Diagnosis		
Respiratory support		
Medical treatment		
Long-term outcome		

CASE STUDIES

Case 1

A 27-year-old woman was admitted from her physician's office following complaints of fatigue. Upon interview, the patient reports that she becomes weak after any exertion, especially in her arms. She also complains of difficulty swallowing. She denies any recent illness. Vital signs show a normal temperature and slightly increased heart rate and respiration. Inspection reveals that she has drooping eyelids and appears to have little tone in her facial muscles.

38. Based on this information, what is the most likely diagnosis?

_____

_____

Copyright © 2025, Elsevier, Inc. All rights reserved.

Chapter **33** **Neuromuscular and Other Diseases of the Chest Wall**

39. What drug therapy might help to confirm this diagnosis?

_____

_____

40. Why is measurement of inspiratory and expiratory pressures a more sensitive test of muscle function than measurement of vital capacity?

Case 2

A 52-year-old man was admitted from his physician's office following complaints of fatigue. Upon interview, he reports that his feet felt numb yesterday and that his legs were weak when he got up this morning. He went to the physician because he thought he might be having a stroke. He states that he had the flu about 2 weeks earlier. Vital signs show a normal temperature and slightly increased heart rate and respiration.

41. Based on this information, what neuromuscular condition is likely?

_____

_____

42. What two treatment strategies have improved outcome in this syndrome?

A. _____

B. _____

WHAT DOES THE NBRC SAY?

Circle the best answer.

43. A 23-year-old patient with flail chest is transferred to the ICU for observation following a motor vehicle accident. After 2 hours, the patient complains of increasing dyspnea, and arterial blood gas analysis is performed.

pH	7.27
$PaCO_2$	55 mm Hg
PaO_2	61 mm Hg

What action should the respiratory therapist recommend at this time?
A. Place the patient on oxygen therapy.
B. Initiate mask CPAP.
C. Administer a bronchodilator drug.
D. Initiate mechanical ventilation.

44. A patient with Guillain-Barré syndrome has had serial vital capacity measurements.

0900	3.1 L
1100	2.6 L
1300	2.1 L
1500	1.6 L

In regard to these data, what should the respiratory therapist recommend?
A. Increase the monitoring to every hour.
B. Administer Tensilon.
C. Provide intubation and mechanical ventilation.
D. Continue to monitor the patient every 2 hours.

Copyright © 2025, Elsevier, Inc. All rights reserved.

45. A vital capacity below what value indicates the need for intubation and ventilation in a patient with acute neuromuscular disease?
   A. 30 ml/kg
   B. 20 ml/kg
   C. 15 ml/kg
   D. 10 ml/kg

46. A patient with myasthenia gravis presents in the emergency department with profound muscle weakness. Administration of which of the following will improve ventilation?
   A. Vecuronium
   B. Neostigmine
   C. Epinephrine
   D. Atropine

47. The presence of paradoxical chest motion on inspiration following a motor vehicle accident most likely indicates

   _____.

   A. flail chest
   B. pulmonary contusion
   C. pneumothorax
   D. hypoxemia

48. A respiratory therapist is assessing a patient in a vegetative state following a stroke. The patient has a pulse of 126 and an SpO_2 of 83% with a tracheostomy collar at 28% oxygen. The therapist attempts to pass a suction catheter but is unsuccessful. What should the therapist do first?
   A. Increase the suction pressure.
   B. Increase the oxygen to 44%.
   C. Initiate mechanical ventilation.
   D. Replace the tracheostomy tube.

FOOD FOR THOUGHT

49. ALS is a disease that strikes down heroes in the prime of life. Prognosis is poor. A newly approved therapy for ALS is riluzole and edaravone. Please discuss these medications in comparison with NIV.

Copyright © 2025, Elsevier, Inc. All rights reserved.

34 Disorders of Sleep

WORD WIZARD

Give the full name of the following acronyms.

1. BiPAP: _____

2. CSA: _____

3. CPAP: _____

4. RDI: _____

5. EEG: _____

6. EPAP: _____

7. IPAP: _____

8. OSA: _____

9. PSG: _____

10. UPPP: _____

11. AHI: _____

MEET THE OBJECTIVES

12. What is the definition of sleep apnea? What about hypopnea?

13. Explain how OSA differs from CSA.

Copyright © 2025, Elsevier, Inc. All rights reserved.

14. What is the estimated incidence of OSA in the adult population?

_____

15. Why does airway closure occur during sleep?

16. List five adverse cardiopulmonary consequences of untreated OSA.

    A. _____

    B. _____

    C. _____

    D. _____

    E. _____

17. List two neurobehavioral and two metabolic consequences of untreated OSA.

    Neurobehavioral

    A. _____

    B. _____

    Metabolic

    C. _____

    D. _____

18. List three factors that predispose a patient to OSA.

    A. _____

    B. _____

    C. _____

19. Describe the six common clinical features seen in many cases of OSA.

    A. _____

    B. _____

    C. _____

    D. _____

    E. _____

    F. _____

20. What is the current gold standard for making a diagnosis of OSA?

_____

Copyright © 2025, Elsevier, Inc. All rights reserved.

21. What value of the apnea-hypopnea index is consistent with moderate to severe sleep apnea? What is considered normal?

22. What are the three goals of treatment for OSA?

A. _____

B. _____

C. _____

23. Discuss the behavioral options that should be pursued in all patients with sleep-disordered breathing.

24. Why do you think nocturnal CPAP has become the first-line medical therapy for OSA?

25. How does CPAP work to relieve OSA?

26. What is auto-titrating CPAP?

Copyright © 2025, Elsevier, Inc. All rights reserved.

27. Identify the indications and explain how the titration of bilevel positive airway pressure therapy differs from that of CPAP.

28. Describe five of the common minor side effects of positive-pressure therapy. Identify what you can do to help the patient solve these annoying problems.

A. _____

B. _____

C. _____

D. _____

E. _____

29. What is the role of tracheostomy in treating sleep apnea?

30. What is the success rate of UPPP, and what is the current recommendation regarding this procedure as a treatment for OSA?

SUMMARY CHECKLIST

Identify the key points from Chapter 33.

31. What are the three types of sleep apnea?

Copyright © 2025, Elsevier, Inc. All rights reserved.

32. What is upper airway stimulation?

33. List two long-term adverse consequences of OSA.

   _____

   _____

34. List two risk factors for OSA.

35. What is the first-line medical therapy for OSA?

36. What therapy may be useful in salvaging patients who have difficulty complying with CPAP?

37. What type of therapy may be an option for a select group of patients who have undergone extensive upper airway analysis and do comply with medical therapy?

   Copyright © 2025, Elsevier, Inc. All rights reserved.

Circle the best answer.

38. An RT notes in the medical record that a patient is receiving BiPAP therapy with a machine he brought from home. Which of the following is the most likely diagnosis for the patient?
    A. Pulmonary emphysema
    B. Congestive heart failure
    C. Obstructive sleep apnea
    D. Central sleep apnea

39. A sleep study shows simultaneous cessation of airflow and respiratory muscle effort. These findings are consistent with _____.
    A. pulmonary hypertension
    B. obstructive sleep apnea
    C. congestive heart failure
    D. central sleep apnea

40. Which of the following is *true* regarding BiPAP therapy?
    1. Expiratory pressure is always set above inspiratory pressure.
    2. BiPAP units are pneumatically powered.
    3. BiPAP should be increased until snoring ceases.
       A. 1 and 3
       B. 2 only
       C. 2 and 3
       D. 3 only

FOOD FOR THOUGHT

If you want to gain more professional expertise on this subject, look no further than the journal *Respiratory Care*, which has editions devoted only to sleep-disordered breathing!

Copyright © 2025, Elsevier, Inc. All rights reserved.

35 Neonatal and Pediatric Respiratory Disorders

WORD WIZARD

Try this matching exercise to test your ability to understand the new terms and acronyms.

Terms	Definitions
_____ 1. MAS	A. Poor clearance of lung fluids
_____ 2. Croup	B. Aspiration of fetal feces
_____ 3. GERD	C. Chronic problem from alveolar trauma and oxygen toxicity
_____ 4. PPHN	D. Life-threatening upper airway infection
_____ 5. MAS	E. Virus-induced subglottic swelling
_____ 6. TTN	F. Acute infection of the lower airways
_____ 7. SIDS	G. Leading cause of death in infants <1 year old
_____ 8. Epiglottitis	H. Complex syndrome of newborn hypertension
_____ 9. BPD	I. Stomach problem associated with asthma
_____ 10. Bronchiolitis	J. A disease in term and near-term infants

BABY BLUES

11. What is the leading cause of death in premature infants?

   _____

12. What is the primary pathophysiology in infants with RDS?

   _____

   _____

13. Describe the four clinical signs of RDS that are listed below.

   A. Respiratory rate: _____

   B. Breathing pattern: _____

   C. Auscultation: _____

   D. Audible sounds: _____

Copyright © 2025, Elsevier, Inc. All rights reserved.

14. How is a definitive diagnosis or RDS usually made?

15. Discuss the four main therapies for treating RDS.
    A. CPAP: Starting values? Device?

    B. Ventilator: When do you start? What is the goal of PEEP for this baby?

    C. Surfactant: When to give? Positioning?

    D. HFV: What does this acronym mean?

Copyright © 2025, Elsevier, Inc. All rights reserved.

16. How does the chest radiograph of a baby with transient tachypnea of the newborn (TTN) differ from that of primary RDS?

17. List two typical respiratory treatments for TTN.

    A. _____

    B. _____

18. Meconium aspiration is usually associated with what fetal event?

    _____

19. MAS usually occurs in infants of what age??

    _____

20. Name the three primary problems in MAS.

    A. _____

    B. _____

    C. _____

21. Describe how air-trapping and barotrauma can occur in an infant with MAS.

22. In some ways, bronchopulmonary dysplasia is a result of our efforts to save preterm infants. What are the five events implicated in causing BPD?

    A. _____

    B. _____

    C. _____

    D. _____

    E. _____

23. What is the "best management" of BPD, and how and where does this begin?

    A. Best: _____

    B. How: _____

    C. Where: _____

218

Copyright © 2025, Elsevier, Inc. All rights reserved.

24. Please define "periodic breathing," and compare that to "abnormal apneic spells."
    A. Periodic breathing:

    B. Abnormal apneic spells:

25. Describe how the following strategies work to alleviate infant apneic events.
    A. Tactile stimulation:

    B. CPAP:

    C. Caffeine (xanthines):

    D. Doxapram (Dopram):

    E. Transfusion:

Copyright © 2025, Elsevier, Inc. All rights reserved.

26. Describe the basic idea behind each of these treatments for PPHN.

    A. Oxygen

    B. Glucose

    C. Inotropes

    D. Sedation

    E. HFV

    F. Inhaled NO

    G. ECMO

27. List the four defects seen in tetralogy of Fallot.

    A. _____

    B. _____

    C. _____

    D. _____

Copyright © 2025, Elsevier, Inc. All rights reserved.

28. Acyanotic heart diseases are also seen in newborns. PDA is of special interest to RTs. Describe PDA. Name two treatments.

A. Description:

B. Treatments:

C. Explain the use of two pulse oximeters in this situation. You'll need to look back at PPHN to find the answer.

PEDIATRIC PROBLEMS

29. Describe the typical profile of a baby who dies of SIDS.

_____

_____

30. What sleeping position is strongly linked with SIDS?

_____

31. Identify the six infant characteristics often seen near the time of death.

A. _____

B. _____

C. _____

D. _____

E. _____

F. _____

32. What is gastroesophageal reflux disease (GERD)? Name a few of the many respiratory problems this condition can trigger.

Copyright © 2025, Elsevier, Inc. All rights reserved.

33. What age group of kids typically develops bronchiolitis?

_____

34. RSV is one particularly nasty virus that's the culprit in many cases of bronchiolitis. Discuss:
    A. Immunization. Who gets it?

    _____

    B. What does RSV stand for?

    _____

    C. How is the diagnosis made?

    _____

35. Dyspnea, tachypnea, wheezing, and cough are common in these kids. If they have to be hospitalized, what respiratory treatments are indicated?
    A. Bronchodilators, recommended or not recommended? _____
    B. Why give antibiotics for a virus? _____
    C. Hygiene? _____

CASE STUDIES

Case 1

A mother brings her previously healthy 1-year-old to the ED. She states that her baby had a cold 2 days ago, but he still has a slight fever and has been coughing. Mom became concerned when she heard audible wheezing. A treatment with albuterol in the ED has had no effect. Vital signs are essentially normal, except for a slight elevation in respiratory rate. The chest radiograph shows mild hyperinflation with no signs of consolidation. Pulse oximetry shows a saturation of 94%.

36. What diagnosis is most likely?

_____

37. How can a diagnosis of RSV be ruled out?

_____

38. The physician decides to send mom and baby home. What treatment would you recommend?

Copyright © 2025, Elsevier, Inc. All rights reserved.

Case 2

A 3-year-old is brought to the ED with respiratory distress and a barking cough. The child has been sick for several days with a low-grade fever and stuffy nose. Examination reveals moderate inspiratory stridor and retractions. The pulse oximeter shows a saturation of 88% on room air. A lateral neck film identifies subglottic narrowing with a "steeple sign."

39. What is the most likely diagnosis?

   _____

40. What aerosolized medication is traditionally delivered?

41. When should you add nebulized budesonide?

42. How would you deliver oxygen to this child?

   _____

Case 3

A 5-year-old is brought to the Emergency Department with labored breathing and a high fever. Examination reveals marked inspiratory stridor. The child is listless, and dad says he has had a sore throat. When you talk to the boy, he responds very quietly with short answers. A lateral neck radiograph identifies a "thumb sign."

43. What is the most likely diagnosis?

   _____

44. What organism is usually responsible for this condition? How could you confirm?

   _____

45. What is the immediate treatment for this condition? Who should perform the intervention and where?

   _____

46. What should not be done? _____

Copyright © 2025, Elsevier, Inc. All rights reserved.

A grandmother brings her son's 2-year-old to the clinic because "his breathing just isn't right." She states, "This boy is coughing all the time. Besides, he isn't growing very well, and when I kiss him, his skin tastes salty!"

47. How would your diagnosis be confirmed? What values indicate CF?

_____

48. What dietary modifications are needed in cystic fibrosis?

_____

49. List four respiratory treatments aimed at decreasing airway obstruction.

A. _____

B. _____

C. _____

D. _____

50. Nebulizing drugs are one of the key treatments in this situation. Tell me more about:
A. Mucolytic drugs:

B. 7% solution:

C. What are tobramycin and aztreonam?

WHAT DOES THE NBRC SAY?

Circle the best answer.

51. A premature infant is experiencing episodes of apnea and cyanosis. The respiratory therapist should recommend which of the following?
A. Albuterol
B. Narcan
C. Exosurf
D. Caffeine

Copyright © 2025, Elsevier, Inc. All rights reserved.

52. A 5-year-old child presents in the ED with complaints of a severe sore throat. The child has inspiratory stridor and muffled phonation. He has a fever of 40°C. His mother states he will not drink anything, so she brought him in.

   The most likely diagnosis is _____.
   A. croup
   B. bronchiolitis
   C. foreign body aspiration
   D. epiglottitis

53. Which of the following tests is helpful in establishing a diagnosis of cystic fibrosis?
   A. Sweat chloride
   B. L/S ratio
   C. Apgar score
   D. Pneumogram

54. Which of the following is the most appropriate imaging technique to help confirm a diagnosis of croup?
   A. Computed tomogram
   B. PA chest film
   C. Lateral neck film
   D. Bronchogram

55. A 4-year-old child with LTB presents in the ED with moderate stridor and harsh breath sounds. The RT should recommend which of the following?
   A. Albuterol
   B. Racemic epinephrine
   C. Immediate intubation
   D. Aminophylline

FOOD FOR THOUGHT

56. What are BRUEs? What are some things that may be observed in infants experiencing and event?

Copyright © 2025, Elsevier, Inc. All rights reserved.

36 Airway Pharmacology

WORD WIZARD

Try this matching exercise to test your ability to understand the new terms found in Chapter 36. (You may have to really dig for some of these—use the chapter, the glossary, and a medical dictionary if necessary!)

Terms	Definitions
1. _____ Indication	A. Time it takes to metabolize half of a drug dose.
2. _____ Tolerance	B. Drug may not be given for any reason
3. _____ Adrenergic	C. Effect of acetylcholine on smooth muscle.
4. _____ Vasopressor	D. Reason for giving a drug to a patient.
5. _____ Prodrug	E. Undesired effect of a drug.
6. _____ Muscarinic	F. Drugs that mimic the effect of epinephrine.
7. _____ Pharmacodynamic	G. Has receptor affinity and exerts an effect.
8. _____ Side effect	H. Mimics the effect of acetylcholine.
9. _____ Absolute contraindication	I. Drug that exerts a constricting effect on blood vessels.
10. _____ Leukotriene	J. Given in an inactive form that converts to active in the body.
11. _____ Mydriasis	K. Dilation of the pupil of the eye.
12. _____ Agonist	L. Phase related to mechanism of action.
13. _____ Pharmacokinetic	M. Maximum effect from a drug dose.
14. _____ Cholinergic	N. Time it takes a drug to start working.
15. _____ Antagonist	O. How long a drug's effect lasts.
16. _____ Tachyphylaxis	P. Increasing dose needed for effect.
17. _____ Onset	Q. Has receptor affinity but produces no effect.
18. _____ Peak effect	R. Rapidly developing tolerance.
19. _____ Duration	S. Compounds that produce allergic or inflammatory responses.
20. _____ Half-life	T. Phase related to metabolism of a drug.

Copyright © 2025, Elsevier, Inc. All rights reserved.

JUST SAY YES

21. What is the most common medication route of administration that is used by RTs?

_____

22. List four advantages of this route.

A. _____

B. _____

C. _____

D. _____

23. List two disadvantages of this route.

A. _____

B. _____

24. How do medications delivered by this route usually end up in the systemic circulation?

_____

25. Describe the two primary divisions of the autonomic nervous system in terms of name, main neurotransmitter, and effect on bronchial smooth muscle.

	DIVISION	OTHER NAME	NEUROTRANSMITTER	AIRWAY MUSCLE EFFECT
A.	Sympathetic			
B.	Parasympathetic			

ADRENERGIC BRONCHODILATORS

26. State the three receptors of the sympathetic nervous system and their basic effects.

	RECEPTOR	PRIMARY EFFECT
A.		
B.		
C.		

Copyright © 2025, Elsevier, Inc. All rights reserved.

27. Give the generic name, brand name, strength, and dose for the following commonly used beta-adrenergic bronchodilators.

	GENERIC NAME	BRAND NAME	STRENGTH	DOSE
A.	Albuterol SVN			
	Albuterol MDI			
	Albuterol DPI			
B.	Levalbuterol SVN			
	Levalbuterol MDI			
C.	Salmeterol DPI			
D.	Formoterol SVN			
E.	Arformoterol SVN			
F.	Olodaterol DPI			

28. It is especially important that you know how long it takes for a drug to start working and reach its maximum effect and how long the drug will last. Fill in the information for the drugs listed below.

	DRUG	ONSET	PEAK EFFECT	DURATION
A.	Xopenex			
B.	Racemic epinephrine			
C.	Proventil			
D.	Serevent			
E.	Formoterol			
F.	Arformoterol			

29. List the most common side effects of bronchodilator drugs. Which one is the most frequent?

A. _____

B. _____

C. _____

D. _____

30. What vital signs should you monitor when administering any drugs via the aerosol route?

A. _____

B. _____

C. _____

D. _____

E. _____

Copyright © 2025, Elsevier, Inc. All rights reserved.

31. How would you assess long-term bronchodilator use?

A. _____

B. _____

C. _____

D. _____

E. _____

ANTICHOLINERGIC BRONCHODILATORS

32. Generally, ipratropium bromide is indicated for use in patients with what pathology?

_____

33. Fill in the blanks to complete your knowledge of anticholinergic medications and combinations of it with SABA and LABA.

DRUG	BRAND NAME	ADULT DOSAGE	TIME COURSE (ONSET, PEAK, DURATION)
Ipratropium bromide			*Onset:* *Peak:* *Duration:*
Ipratropium bromide and albuterol			*Onset:* *Peak:* *Duration:*
Aclidinium bromide			*Onset:* *Peak:* *Duration:*
Aclidinium bromide and formoterol			*Onset:* *Peak:* *Duration:*
Glycopyrrolate bromide			*Onset:* *Peak:* *Duration:*
Glycopyrrolate bromide and formoterol			*Onset:* *Peak:* *Duration:*
Glycopyrrolate bromide and formoterol			*Onset:* *Peak:* *Duration:*

Copyright © 2025, Elsevier, Inc. All rights reserved.

DRUG	BRAND NAME	ADULT DOSAGE	TIME COURSE (ONSET, PEAK, DURATION)
Revefenacin			*Onset:* *Peak:* *Duration:*
Tiotropium bromide			*Onset:* *Peak:* *Duration:*
Tiotropium bromide and olodaterol			*Onset:* *Peak:* *Duration:*

34. Describe the side effects to watch for when administering this class of drugs.
Common side effects

A. _____

B. _____

MDI occasional side effects

A. _____

B. _____

SVN occasional side effects

A. _____

B. _____

MUCUS CONTROLLING AGENTS

35. Describe the mucoactive agents available for nebulization.

	AGENT	BRAND NAME	DOSE	INDICATION
A.	Acetylcysteine 10% or 20%			
B.	Dornase alfa			
C.	Aqueous water, saline			
D.	Hyperosmolar 3-7% saline			
E.	Mannitol			

36. Bronchospasm is a common side effect of the administration of mucolytic agents. How would you recommend modifying the therapy to prevent or treat this problem?

Copyright © 2025, Elsevier, Inc. All rights reserved.

37. What types of short-term and long-term assessments should you make to monitor the effectiveness of these drugs?

INHALED CORTICOSTEROIDS

38. How long will it take for inhaled steroids to have a noticeable effect on the symptoms of asthma?

39. What significance does this have in terms of patient education?

40. The most common side effects of inhaled steroids are local ones (as opposed to systemic). Name the four most common problems.

A. _____

B. _____

C. _____

D. _____

41. Fill in the blanks to complete your knowledge of Corticosteroids and combination products.

Drug	Brand Name(s)	Formulation and Dosage
Beclomethasone dipropionate		
Ciclesonide		
Fluticasone propionate		
Fluticasone furoate		
Budesonide		
Mometasone furoate		
Fluticasone propionate/salmeterol		
Budesonide/formoterol fumarate HFA		
Mometasone furoate/formoterol fumarate HFA		
Fluticasone furoate/vilanterol		
Fluticasone furoate/umeclidinium/vilanterol		
Budesonide/glycopyrrolate/ formoterol		

Copyright © 2025, Elsevier, Inc. All rights reserved.

42. What would you assess to determine if the steroids were working in the long run?

_____

NONSTEROIDAL ANTIASTHMA DRUGS

43. What is dupilumab? What patient population may benefit from this medication?

_____

44. List the number one side effect for each of the following:

A. Zafirlukast(Accolate): _____

B. Zileuton (Zyflo): _____

C. Montelukast(Singulair): _____

TREATING INFECTION BY THE AEROSOL ROUTE

45. What agent may be nebulized to treat *P. jiroveci* seen in severely immunocompromised patients?

_____

46. What are the common undesired respiratory side effects of administration? What modification of therapy would you recommend if they occur?

_____

47. While *P. jiroveci* is not a hazard to healthy people, patients with AIDS often have what other disease that is transmitted via the airborne route?

_____

48. Describe the use of ribavirin in terms of indication, patient population, and special equipment needed for administration.

A. Indication: _____

B. Type of patient: _____

C. Nebulizer: _____

D. Organism: _____

49. What about TOBI?

A. Drug: _____

B. Type of patient: _____

C. Nebulizer: _____

D. Organism: _____

50. What about Aztreonam?

A. Drug: _____

B. Type of patient: _____

C. Nebulizer: _____

D. Organism: _____

233

Copyright © 2025, Elsevier, Inc. All rights reserved.

INFLUENZA

51. Which inhaled drug can shorten the course of influenza and alleviate symptoms? What is the problem with giving it to asthma and COPD patients?

    A. Drug: _____

    B. Problem: _____

    C. Delivery system: _____

    D. What is the "off-label use?" _____

INHALED VASODILATORS

52. Specifically, when is nitric oxide used for newborns? When is it contraindicated?

53. What is the most common adverse reaction during weaning from nitric oxide? What type of hemoglobin disorder could be monitored?

54. What is the brand name of iloprost? What is the class of drugs it represents? (Be specific.)

    A. _____

    B. _____

55. What nebulizer is used to deliver the drug?

56. Describe treprostinil.

    A. Indications and goal: _____

    B. Delivery system: _____

    C. Mode of action: _____

Copyright © 2025, Elsevier, Inc. All rights reserved.

Case 1

A patient who has asthma is admitted to the hospital for the second time in 2 months. She has not been able to get relief and is using her albuterol inhaler frequently.

57. In addition to inhaled beta agonists, steroids are commonly administered to *reduce* inflammation associated with asthma. Name one inhaled steroid and recommend a dosage.

58. What device is important to use along with MDIs to prevent deposition of these drugs in the mouth?

59. Why should this patient rinse her mouth after use of her inhaled steroid?

60. What long-acting bronchodilator may help this patient sleep through the night without being awakened by dyspnea and wheezing?

Case 2

Cystic fibrosis is diagnosed in a 7-year-old. This patient has extremely thick mucus (like glue!). Auscultation reveals scattered wheezing and rhonchi.

61. What drug would you recommend aerosolizing for treatment of the thick mucus?

62. What other drug should be given to treat the wheezing?

63. He has *Pseudomonas* in his sputum. What could you nebulize to treat gram-negative bad boys in CF?

Case 3

A 67-year-old man with long-standing COPD characterized by chronic bronchitis is coughing up copious amounts of very thick white sputum. He complains that his chest feels tight, and he cannot catch his breath. His albuterol inhaler is not providing relief.

64. What bronchodilator is appropriate to add to the therapeutic regimen?

65. What alternative delivery methods might be useful?

Copyright © 2025, Elsevier, Inc. All rights reserved.

A respiratory care student is administering a standard dose of albuterol via SVN to a 65-year-old male admitted for pneumonia and COPD. Five minutes into the treatment the patient's heart rate increases from 92 to 156 on the monitor. The instructor walks in at this moment.

66. What action should the student do first? What other actions might be taken right away at the bedside?

67. What diagnostic test should be ordered?

68. What change in medication could provide bronchodilation with fewer side effects?

WHAT DOES THE NBRC SAY?

Try these exercises. Circle the best answer.

69. A patient with asthma comes to the emergency department with dyspnea, hypoxemia, and wheezing. The appropriate
    medication at this time is _____.
    A. administration of nitric oxide
    B. nebulized formoterol (Performist)
    C. nebulized albuterol (Ventolin)
    D. nebulized ipratropium bromide (Atrovent)

70. Following extubation, a patient has mild stridor. Which of the following would you recommend at this time?
    A. Administration of oxygen
    B. Aerosolized albuterol (Proventil)
    C. Aerosolized virazole (Ribavirin)
    D. Aerosolized racemic epinephrine

71. After administering a corticosteroid via MDI, the RT should ask the patient to perform which of the following actions?
    A. Rinse and gargle with water.
    B. Deep breathe and cough.
    C. Inhale an adrenergic bronchodilator.
    D. Inhale via a spacer device.

Copyright © 2025, Elsevier, Inc. All rights reserved.

72. The heart rate of a patient receiving an adrenergic bronchodilator rises from 80 to 94 beats per minute during the treatment. Which of the following actions is most appropriate?
    A. The RT should discontinue the therapy.
    B. Let the patient rest for 5 minutes.
    C. Continue the treatment.
    D. Reduce the dosage of the bronchodilator.

73. A physician calls in an order for bronchodilator therapy for a patient with COPD. The order states, "0.05 ml of

    albuterol in 3 ml of normal saline via SVN four times per day." The RT should _____.
    A. deliver the treatment as ordered
    B. recommend substituting Atrovent
    C. carefully monitor heart rate during the treatment
    D. call the physician to verify the order

74. Which of the following is the most commonly used rescue medication for acute episodes of bronchospasm?
    A. Albuterol
    B. Atrovent
    C. Advair
    D. Tiotropium bromide

FOOD FOR THOUGHT

75. Besides treatment of excessively thick mucus, what else can acetylcysteine be used for?

_____

_____

Copyright © 2025, Elsevier, Inc. All rights reserved.

37 Airway Management

SUCTIONING

1. What is the name of the device commonly used to suction secretions or fluids from the oropharynx?

   _____

2. Describe the cause of and how to prevent each of the following complications.

	COMPLICATION	CAUSE	PREVENTION
A.	Hypoxemia		
B.	Cardiac arrhythmia		
C.	Hypotension		
D.	Atelectasis		
E.	Mucosal trauma		
F.	Increased ICP		
G.	Bacterial colonization of lower airway		

3. Discuss the advantages and disadvantages of in-line suction catheters.
   A. Advantages:

   B. Disadvantages

4. What special catheter is used to facilitate entry into the left mainstem bronchus?

   _____

5. What specialized airway is used to facilitate repeated nasal suctioning?

   _____

6. What device do you need to include when you want to collect a sputum specimen during suctioning?

   _____

238

Copyright © 2025, Elsevier, Inc. All rights reserved.

7. What type of lung disease requires the use of a double-lumen ET tube?

_____

What is the name of the special type of ventilation used with this tube?

_____

8. High-frequency jet ventilation tubes look like standard tubes with two additional lines. What are they?

A. _____

B. _____

9. What is the reported benefit of the subglottic suction tube on specialized ETT?

_____

INTUBATION PROCEDURES

10. What is the preferred route for establishing an emergency tracheal airway?

_____

11. Why is suction equipment needed for intubation?

_____

12. Describe two common troubleshooting procedures used when the laryngoscope does not light up properly.

_____

13. Prior to insertion, how should the RT test the tube?

_____

14. How is the patient's head positioned to align the mouth, pharynx, and larynx?

_____

15. What other actions *must be taken* before making any attempt to intubate?

_____

16. How long should you attempt intubation? Why do you think we have a rule like this one?

_____

17. List at least two anatomic landmarks *in addition to the glottis* that should be visualized prior to intubation.

A. _____

B. _____

18. Compare the use of the Miller and Macintosh laryngoscope blades during the intubation procedure.

Copyright © 2025, Elsevier, Inc. All rights reserved.

19. List nine methods for bedside assessment of correct tube position.

A. _____

B. _____

C. _____

D. _____

E. _____

F. _____

G. _____

H. _____

I. _____

20. What is the disadvantage of using capnographic or colorimetric analysis of carbon dioxide to assess intubation in a cardiac arrest victim?

21. What is the final step of confirmation of endotracheal tube placement?

_____

22. Give two examples of clinical situations where nasotracheal intubation might be preferred over oral intubation.

A. _____

B. _____

23. Describe the two techniques used for nasal intubation.

A. _____

B. _____

24. You may need to use medications to facilitate intubation. What drugs would you use to:

A. Numb the airway and reflexes

B. Sedate the patient

C. Paralyze the patient

Copyright © 2025, Elsevier, Inc. All rights reserved.

TRACHEOTOMY

25. What is the primary indication for performing a tracheotomy?

   _____

   _____

26. Describe the sequence for removing an ET during the tracheotomy procedure.

27. Compare the location of placement in percutaneous and traditional surgical tracheotomy.

28. Name at least three advantages of the percutaneous technique compared with traditional surgical tracheotomy.

   A. _____

   B. _____

   C. _____

AIRWAY TRAUMA

29. Compare the following laryngeal injuries associated with intubation in terms of symptoms and treatment.

	INJURY	SYMPTOMS	TREATMENT
A.	Glottic edema		
B.	Vocal cord inflammation		
C.	Laryngeal ulceration		
D.	Polyp/granuloma		
E.	Vocal cord paralysis		
F.	Laryngeal stenosis		

30. Describe the tracheoesophageal fistula in terms of cause, complications, and treatment.

Copyright © 2025, Elsevier, Inc. All rights reserved.

31. Tracheoinnominate artery fistula is a rare but serious complication. What are the clues, and what are the immediate and corrective actions to take?

What is the survival rate?

CARE OF AN ARTIFICIAL AIRWAY

32. What is the most common material used to secure endotracheal tubes? Tracheostomy tubes?

_____

What is the alternative?

_____

33. How do flexion and extension of the neck affect tube motion? What is the average distance the tube will move (in cm)?

34. What is a "talking" trach? What are some of the problems with these devices?

35. When using a Passy-Muir Valve, what do you need to do with the cuff? How about the ventilator?

HUMIDIFICATION

36. What is the worst problem that results from inadequate humidification of the artificial airway?

_____

242

Copyright © 2025, Elsevier, Inc. All rights reserved.

37. What temperature range must be maintained in a heated humidification system to provide adequate inspired moisture?

_____

38. What device can be used as an alternative to heated humidifiers for short-term humidification of the intubated patient?

_____

39. What is the most common cause of airway obstruction in the critically ill patient?

_____

CUFF CARE

40. What is the recommended safe cuff pressure? What is the consequence of elevated cuff pressures?

41. What may happen when the tube is too small for the patient's trachea?

_____

TRACH CARE

42. Briefly describe the eight basic steps of tracheotomy care.

A. _____

B. _____

C. _____

D. _____

E. _____

F. _____

G. _____

H. _____

AIRWAY EMERGENCIES

43. List three airway emergencies.

A. _____

B. _____

C. _____

Copyright © 2025, Elsevier, Inc. All rights reserved.

44. List four possible reasons why a tube may become obstructed.

A. _____

B. _____

C. _____

D. _____

45. What simple technique is used to assess tube obstructions that are not relieved by repositioning the head or deflating the cuff?

_____

46. If you cannot clear the obstruction, what action should you be prepared to take?

_____

47. What additional troubleshooting step can often be performed on patients with tracheostomies?

_____

48. What effects will occur with a cuff leak when a patient is being mechanically ventilated?

_____

EXTUBATION AND DECANNULATION

49. The decision to remove the airway and the decision to remove the ventilator are not the same. What kind of patients might need to remain intubated even after the ventilator is removed?

_____

50. Describe the method for performing a "cuff-leak test."
    What does *Egan's* suggest as a percentage of leak that should lead to considering extubation?

51. List five types of equipment you will want to assemble *prior* to extubation.

A. _____

B. _____

C. _____

D. _____

E. _____

52. What therapeutic modality is usually applied immediately after extubation?

_____

Copyright © 2025, Elsevier, Inc. All rights reserved.

53. List three of the most common problems that occur after extubation.

54. A common complication of extubation is glottic edema. How will you recognize *and* treat this problem?

55. List three methods for weaning from a tracheostomy tube. Give one advantage and one disadvantage for each technique. This is national exam material.

	TECHNIQUE	ADVANTAGE	DISADVANTAGE
A.			
B.			
C.			

AIRWAY ALTERNATIVES

56. List three advantages of the LMA.

A. _____

B. _____

C. _____

57. List two disadvantages of the LMA.

A. _____

B. _____

CASE STUDIES

Case 1

During your first day of clinical training in the ICU, a patient sustains a cardiac arrest. Your clinical instructor asks you to assist in preparing the equipment needed for endotracheal intubation. The patient is a small 56-year-old female.

58. What size endotracheal tube should you select?

_____

59. How should you test the tube prior to insertion?

_____

60. How will you test the laryngoscope and blade for proper function?

_____

245

Copyright © 2025, Elsevier, Inc. All rights reserved.

61. Once the tube is inserted, how can you quickly assess placement?

Case 2

After your heart-pounding initiation into resuscitation, it is time to check the other ventilator patients in the unit. A 19-year-old woman with a head injury is receiving mechanical ventilation via a cuffed No. 8 tracheostomy tube with an inner cannula. As you enter the room, the high-pressure alarm is sounding.

62. How will you determine the need for suctioning in this situation?

___

63. What vacuum pressure should be set prior to suctioning?

___

64. What size suction catheter is suggested?

___

65. What F_IO_2 should you preoxygenate this patient?

___

WHAT DOES THE NBRC SAY?

Circle the best answer.

66. Which of the following will decrease the risk of damage to the trachea from the endotracheal tube cuff?
    1. Inflating the cuff with less than 10 ml air
    2. Maintaining cuff pressures of 25 cm H_2O
    3. Using a high-volume low-pressure cuff
    4. Inflating the cuff to 25-35 mm Hg
        A. 1 and 2
        B. 1 and 3
        C. 2 and 3
        D. 3 and 4

67. The diameter of the suction catheter for an adult should be no larger than
    A. one-tenth the inner diameter of the ET tube.
    B. one-third the inner diameter of the ET tube.
    C. one-half the inner diameter of the ET tube.
    D. three-fourths the inner diameter of the ET tube.

68. Extubation is performed on a patient with an endotracheal tube. Presence of which of the following suggests the presence of upper airway edema?
    A. Rhonchi
    B. Crackles
    C. Wheezes
    D. Stridor

69. Which of the following tools is not needed during nasotracheal intubation?
    A. Laryngoscope handle
    B. Stylette
    C. Miller blade
    D. Magill forceps

Copyright © 2025, Elsevier, Inc. All rights reserved.

70. While performing endotracheal suctioning, an RT notes that flow-through is minimal and secretion clearance is sluggish. Which of the following are possible causes of this problem?
    1. The vacuum setting is greater than 120 mm Hg.
    2. The suction canister is full of secretions.
    3. There is a leak in the system.
    4. The tube cuff is overinflated.
    A. 1 and 2
    B. 1 and 4
    C. 2 and 3
    D. 3 and 4

71. Rapid, initial determination of endotracheal tube placement can be achieved by _____.
    1. auscultation
    2. arterial blood gas analysis
    3. measurement of end-tidal CO_2
    4. measurement of SpO_2
    A. 1 and 2
    B. 1 and 3
    C. 2 and 4
    D. 3 and 4

72. A patient with a tracheostomy tube shows signs of severe airway obstruction. A suction catheter will pass only a short distance into the tube. The RT should _____.
    A. remove the tracheostomy tube
    B. inflate the cuff of the tube
    C. ventilate the tube with positive pressure
    D. remove the inner cannula

73. Which of the following can be used to assess pulmonary circulation during closed-chest cardiac compressions?
    A. Capnometry
    B. Arterial blood gas analysis
    C. Pulse oximetry
    D. Blood pressure monitoring

74. Prior to performing bronchoscopy, an RT is asked to administer a nebulized anesthetic to the patient. What medication is most appropriate to place in the nebulizer?
    A. Versed
    B. Atropine
    C. Morphine
    D. Lidocaine

FOOD FOR THOUGHT

75. Following emergency cricothyroidotomy, when should a definitive airway be established?

Copyright © 2025, Elsevier, Inc. All rights reserved.

38 Emergency Cardiovascular Life Support

Write out the full definition of each acronym below.

1. CABD: _____

2. ACLS: _____

3. AED: _____

4. AHA: _____

5. BLS: _____

6. SCA: _____

7. CDC: _____

8. CNS: _____

9. CPR: _____

10. FBAO: _____

11. EMS: _____

12. PALS: _____

CAUSES AND PREVENTION OF SUDDEN DEATH

13. What is the primary cause of sudden death in the United States?

_____

14. What is the most common rhythm immediately after cardiac arrest? Briefly describe the two basic treatments.

A. Rhythm: _____

B. Treatments: _____

_____

Copyright © 2025, Elsevier, Inc. All rights reserved.

15. Compare adult, child, and infant resuscitation for the following categories for two rescuers.

	CATEGORY	ADULT	CHILD	INFANT
A.	Compression 1. Hand placement 2. Depth 3. Rate 4. Where to check pulse			
B.	Obstructed airway 1. Responsive 2. Unresponsive			
C.	Ventilation 1. Rate 2. Ratio			

16. You wouldn't want to do CPR on someone who is just sedated. Once you carefully assess unresponsiveness, you need HELP! What should you do in each of these situations?
    A. Collapsed outside hospital:

    _____

    B. In the hospital:

    _____

    C. How do you quickly check for "signs of life?"

    _____

    _____

17. When is the jaw-thrust maneuver indicated?

    _____

18. How is assessment of pulselessness different in adults and infants?

19. Once CPR is begun, it is normally only stopped for what three reasons?

    A. _____

    B. _____

    C. _____

Copyright © 2025, Elsevier, Inc. All rights reserved.

DEFIBRILLATION

20. What is the most likely rhythm of a person with sudden cardiac arrest?

    _____

21. Why is early defibrillation so important?

    _____

22. Describe the AED briefly. Is the shock really automatic? After hooking up the electrodes, what else is the operator supposed to do?

YES, BUT IS IT GOOD CPR?

23. How can you easily and quickly determine the effectiveness of ventilations and compressions delivered during CPR?

    A. Ventilation: _____

    B. Compression: _____

24. CPR can have complications. State a way to avoid these classics.

    A. Neck injury: _____

    B. Gastric inflation: _____

    C. Vomiting: _____

    D. Internal trauma (liver laceration): _____

    E. FBAO removal: _____

25. CPR is contraindicated under what two circumstances?

    A. _____

    B. _____

26. What barriers does the CDC suggest to protect us during CPR?

    _____

FOREIGN BODIES

27. What is the universal distress signal for foreign body obstruction of the airway?

    _____

250

Copyright © 2025, Elsevier, Inc. All rights reserved.

28. Give another name for the abdominal thrust maneuver.

_____

When should you avoid this maneuver in an adult?

_____

What should you do if you cannot or should not perform the abdominal thrust on a choking victim?

29. Describe four ways you can use to determine if the foreign body has been removed from the airway.

A. _____

B. _____

C. _____

D. _____

ADVANCED CARDIAC LIFE SUPPORT

30. What concentration of oxygen should be administered during a life-threatening emergency?

_____

31. What is the technique to select the best-sized oropharyngeal airway (OPA)?

32. What airway would you choose for the patient who cannot tolerate an oral airway?

_____

33. Describe two ways to insert an oral airway without pushing the tongue back.

A. _____

B. _____

34. When are oropharyngeal airways contraindicated?

_____

35. Why is an endotracheal tube the preferred method for securing the airway during CPR?

Copyright © 2025, Elsevier, Inc. All rights reserved.

36. Describe the proper way to ventilate during resuscitation. Include volumes, rates, ratios—all methods to avoid hyper-inflation and other problems.

37. When should the endotracheal route of drug administration be used?

38. What is the primary treatment for pulseless ventricular tachycardia and ventricular fibrillation?

_____

39. List three medications that can be delivered via the ET route.

A. _____

B. _____

C. _____

40. What modification to dosage and technique must be made for endotracheal instillation of emergency drugs?

_____

41. What initial energy level is recommended for electrical countershock during ventricular fibrillation using a biphasic defibrillator? What about monophasic? How about any subsequent shocks?

42. Explain the difference between cardioversion and defibrillation.

43. When is electrical pacing indicated?

_____

Copyright © 2025, Elsevier, Inc. All rights reserved.

44. Complete the following chart regarding drugs used in advanced cardiovascular life support.

Drug	Indications	Contraindications	Route	Dosage	Pharmacologic Effects
Adenosine					
Amiodarone					
Atropine sulfate					
Dopamine					
Epinephrine					
Isoproterenol					
Lidocaine					
Propranolol					
Verapamil, diltiazem					

CASE STUDIES

Case 1

A man at the corner table is eating and having coffee. Suddenly he puts his hands to his throat and tries to stand. He is unable to cough or speak.

45. What is your first action?

46. How would you remedy the FBAO?

47. If the victim becomes unconscious, how will you modify your technique?

Copyright © 2025, Elsevier, Inc. All rights reserved.

Your coffee is ready, but before you can drink one sip, a red-faced executive-type in a suit collapses to the floor. . .

48. According to "Basic Life Support" guidelines, you need to perform six steps in the right order.
    A. First determine unresponsiveness. What would you check? What would you do?

    B. Step two is checking the _____.
    C. Now you need to call for help. Be specific for this setting.
    D. This victim has become unresponsive and basically dead on the spot. What device do you need right now to assess the heart and treat the most likely rhythm for sudden cardiac arrest?

    E. No devices are available. You need to start _____ at a rate of

    _____.

    F. Open the _____ and check for _____.

    G. He's still dead. You should give two _____.

You are dreaming of your coffee, but the paramedics arrive. They defibrillate the victim and his pulse returns but not his breathing. The paramedics ask for your help with airway management.

49. Select an initial device to manage the airway in an unconscious victim.

50. You must begin ventilation with bag and mask. Of course you use oxygen, but what rate is needed in this case and how long is inhalation?

51. What is the biggest hazard to the patient during bag-mask ventilation?

 Copyright © 2025, Elsevier, Inc. All rights reserved.

Circle the correct answer.

52. When is the jaw-thrust technique indicated to help maintain an airway?
    A. When foreign body obstruction is suspected
    B. In pediatric patients
    C. In cases of suspected neck injury
    D. During most CPR efforts

53. Where should you check the pulse of an unresponsive infant?
    A. Brachial artery
    B. Carotid artery
    C. Femoral artery
    D. Radial artery

54. Upon entering a hospital room, you see a physical therapist administering CPR to a patient who is lying on the floor.

    Your first action would be to _____.
    A. move the patient onto the bed
    B. call for help
    C. take over chest compressions
    D. deliver two slow breaths to the airway

55. An unconscious patient begins gagging during your attempt to insert an oropharyngeal airway. The correct action to

    take at this time would be to _____.
    A. insert a smaller oral airway
    B. intubate the patient
    C. perform the jaw-thrust maneuver
    D. insert a nasal airway

56. The ideal airway to use during a resuscitation effort is a(n) _____.
    A. oropharyngeal airway
    B. nasopharyngeal airway
    C. fenestrated tracheostomy tube
    D. oral endotracheal tube

57. A patient is coughing and wheezing after accidentally aspirating a piece of meat. At this time, the RT should

    _____.
    A. allow the patient to clear his airway
    B. perform the Heimlich maneuver
    C. deliver five back blows
    D. call for help

58. Upon entering an ICU room, an RT observes ventricular fibrillation on the cardiac monitor. The most appropriate

    treatment for this rhythm is _____.
    A. CPR
    B. administration of lidocaine
    C. administration of epinephrine
    D. defibrillation

59. During an adult resuscitation effort, no IV line can be established. The RT should recommend _____.
    A. intramuscular infusion of the medications
    B. endotracheal instillation of the medications
    C. insertion of a central line
    D. aerosol administration of the medications

Copyright © 2025, Elsevier, Inc. All rights reserved.

60. The effectiveness of chest compressions in producing circulation can be measured by _____.
    1. pulse oximetry
    2. capnography
    3. transcutaneous monitoring
    4. arterial blood gases
       A. 1 and 2 only
       B. 2 and 3 only
       C. 2 and 4 only
       D. 1 and 4 only

61. A patient has atrial fibrillation with serious signs and symptoms that do not respond to medications. The treatment of

    choice would be _____.
       A. vagal stimulation
       B. defibrillation
       C. oxygen administration
       D. cardioversion

Get the picture? Any question on the subject of resuscitation is fair game. Start by learning the basic rates, depths, and management techniques. Then move on to the advanced material.

FOOD FOR THOUGHT

62. How can we improve the quality of care given during codes?

63. Who provides emotional support to the family of a resuscitation victim? Who provides support for the health care providers?

64. Are cardioversion and defibrillation the same? If not, how do they differ?

Copyright © 2025, Elsevier, Inc. All rights reserved.

39 Humidity and Bland Aerosol Therapy

Define the following terms.

1. Hygrometer:

2. BTPS conditions:

3. Isothermic saturation boundary:

4. Inspissated:

MEET THE OBJECTIVES

Humidity Therapy

5. Explain inspiration and exhalation as they relate to how gas is heated and humidified under normal conditions.

6. List four factors that can shift the isothermic saturation boundary distally.

   A. _____

   B. _____

   C. _____

   D. _____

7. List four consequences of prolonged inspiration of improperly conditioned gases.

   A. _____

   B. _____

   C. _____

   D. _____

8. Liter flows exceeding what value require humidification?

   _____

9. Give one situation where you would **ALWAYS** provide humidification.

   _____

Copyright © 2025, Elsevier, Inc. All rights reserved.

10. List two indications for humidification.

   A. _____

   B. _____

11. List the four variables that affect the quality of performance of a humidifier.

   A. _____

   B. _____

   C. _____

   D. _____

   Which is most important?

   _____

12. Bubble humidifiers are added to what type of oxygen delivery system?

   _____

13. What is the typical range for absolute humidity delivered by a bubble humidifier? What does this amount convert to in terms of relative body humidity?

   A. Output _____ to _____ mg/L

   B. Relative body humidity = _____%

14. What safety device is incorporated into the design of a bubble humidifier?

   _____

15. Discuss the three primary advantages of passover humidifiers compared with bubble humidifiers.

   A. _____

   B. _____

   C. _____

16. Describe the principle of operation of each of the following heat and moisture exchangers (HMEs).
   A. Simple condenser humidifier:

   B. Hygroscopic condenser humidifier:

   C. Hydrophobic condenser humidifier:

Copyright © 2025, Elsevier, Inc. All rights reserved.

17. List five contraindications to using HMEs, according to the AARC Clinical Practice Guideline on humidification during mechanical ventilation?

A. _____

B. _____

C. _____

D. _____

E. _____

18. What is an "active HME?"

19. Identify three possible risks of using heated humidifiers.

A. _____

B. _____

C. _____

20. Identify three hazards associated with water that "rains out," or condenses, in humidified breathing circuits.

A. _____

B. _____

C. _____

21. List five factors that influence the amount of condensation in a breathing circuit?

A. _____

B. _____

C. _____

D. _____

E. _____

22. What specialized breathing circuit circumvents (usually) the condensation problem?

23. The AARC recommends what range of alarm settings for electronically controlled heated humidifiers?

_____

Copyright © 2025, Elsevier, Inc. All rights reserved.

Bland Aerosols

24. List seven indications given in the AARC Clinical Practice Guidelines for bland aerosol administration.

A. _____

B. _____

C. _____

D. _____

E. _____

F. _____

G. _____

25. What preset variable determines the size of the aerosol particles generated by a USN?

_____

26. What adjustable control determines the actual amount of aerosol produced?

_____

27. Large-volume jet nebulizers are often used to provide moisture to the airway of patients with tracheostomy tubes. When would you use this on a patient who is not intubated?

28. What provides the power to operate a large-volume jet nebulizer?

_____

29. Large-volume jet nebulizers are also useful in controlling F_IO_2. How is this accomplished?

30. Identify the two primary clinical problems associated with tents and body enclosures?

A. _____

B. _____

Copyright © 2025, Elsevier, Inc. All rights reserved.

31. Your text identifies six important problems associated with bland aerosol therapy. For each of these problems, give a possible solution or means of prevention.

Problem	Solution
A. Cross-contamination/infection	_____
B. Environmental safety	_____
C. Inadequate mist	_____
D. Overhydration	_____
E. Bronchospasm	_____
F. Noise	_____

CALCULATIONS

32. At body temperature, gas has a saturated capacity of about 44 mg of water vapor per liter. If a gas has an absolute humidity of 22 mg/L, what is the relative humidity?

Formula _____

Solution _____

Answer _____

33. What is the humidity deficit in Question 32?

Formula _____

Solution _____

Answer _____

SUMMARY CHECKLIST

Complete the following sentences by writing in the correct information in the spaces provided.

34. How is the conditioning of inspired gases is done normally?

35. Gases delivered to the trachea should be warmed between what temperatures?

36. Define a humidifier.

Copyright © 2025, Elsevier, Inc. All rights reserved.

37. Define a nebulizer.

38. What is the most important factor affecting humidifier output.

39. At high flows, what can some bubble humidifiers may produce that may carry infectious bacteria?

40. How should you treat breathing circuit condensate?

CASE STUDIES

Choose the correct humidity or bland aerosol system.

Case 1

A man is brought to the emergency department with a core temperature of 30°C after falling into a lake while ice fishing. The patient is intubated with a No. 8 endotracheal tube. The patient is unconscious and requires mechanical ventilation.

41. Does this patient have any contraindications for HME use?

_____

42. What humidification system would you recommend?

_____

Case 2

A 32-year-old man is admitted to the medical floor with a diagnosis of *Mycoplasma pneumoniae* pneumonia. He is receiving oxygen via nasal cannula at 5 L/min. He complains of a stuffy, dry nose a few hours after admission.

43. What humidification system would you recommend for this patient?

_____

Copyright © 2025, Elsevier, Inc. All rights reserved.

44. Why is this patient unable to benefit from an HME?

_____

Case 3

A 57-year-old man who has undergone coronary artery bypass graft surgery (CABG) is being mechanically ventilated with a No. 8 ET tube pending recovery from the procedure. He has no secretion problems or history of lung problems. Body temperature is normal.

45. What humidification system would you recommend?

_____

46. What signs would you see on chest exam that would tell you that you need to switch this patient to a different device?

_____

WHAT DOES THE NBRC SAY?

Circle the best answer.

47. A respiratory therapist hears a loud whistling sound as she enters the room of a patient receiving oxygen via cannula at 6 L/min. In reference to the humidifier, what is the most likely cause of the problem?
    A. The top of the humidifier is cross-threaded.
    B. The humidifier has run out of water.
    C. The flow rate is set at less than the ordered amount.
    D. There is a kink in the oxygen supply tubing.

48. A USN is ordered for sputum induction. Which of the following solutions should be placed in the medication cup to accomplish this goal?
    A. Sterile distilled water
    B. 0.45% NaCl solution
    C. 0.9% NaCl solution
    D. 3% NaCl solution

49. A large-volume all-purpose nebulizer is set at an F_IO_2 of 0.40 and a flow rate of 10 L/min to deliver humidified oxygen to a patient with a tracheostomy. The nebulizer is producing very little mist. Which of the following could be done to improve the aerosol output?
    1. Check the water level in the nebulizer.
    2. Increase the flow rate to the nebulizer.
    3. Drain condensate from the supply tubing.
    4. Turn off the nebulizer's heating system.
        A. 1 only
        B. 1 and 2 only
        C. 1 and 3 only
        D. 1, 3, and 4 only

50. While performing a ventilator check, the respiratory therapist observes a large amount of thin, white mucus in the tubing connected to the HME. Which of the following actions should be taken at this time?
    A. Rinse out the HME with sterile water.
    B. Suction the mucus from the tubing.
    C. Place the patient on a heated humidification system.
    D. Replace the HME.

Copyright © 2025, Elsevier, Inc. All rights reserved.

Chapter **39** **Humidity and Bland Aerosol Therapy**

51. Sputum induction via USN is ordered. The nebulizer will produce an output of 5 ml of water per minute on the maximum amplitude setting. The treatment is to last for 15 minutes. How much solution should the RCP respiratory therapist place in the nebulizer?
    A. 5 ml
    B. 15 ml
    C. 50 ml
    D. 75 ml

52. Which of the following patients is a greatest risk for overhydration secondary to continuous use of a heated jet nebulizer?
    A. 5-kg infant with croup
    B. 70-year-old COPD patient
    C. 25-year-old patient in need of a sputum induction
    D. 7-year-old asthma patient with pneumonia

FOOD FOR THOUGHT

53. The industry standard for adding simple humidification to an oxygen delivery system is a flow rate of greater than 4 L/min. Can you think of any situations where you might add humidification when the flow rate is lower than 4?

54. What gas flow rate is a HFNC typically set at for adults? Neonates? Pediatrics?

 Copyright © 2025, Elsevier, Inc. All rights reserved.

40 Aerosol Drug Therapy

Match the following terms to their definitions.

Terms	Definitions
1. _____ Aerosol	A. Suspension of solid or liquid particles in a gas.
2. _____ Atomizer	B. Difference between therapeutic and toxic drug concentrations.
3. _____ Baffle	C. Device that produces uniformly sized aerosol particles.
4. _____ Deposition	D. Device that removes large particles
5. _____ Hygroscopic	E. Device that produces non–uniformly sized aerosol particles.
6. _____ Inertial impaction	F. Deposition of particles by collision.
7. _____ MMAD	G. Testimony of a witness (or particles being retained in the respiratory tract!).
8. _____ Nebulizer	H. Absorbs moisture from the air.
9. _____ Propellant	I. Measurement of average particle size
10. _____ Therapeutic index	J. Amount of drug left in the SVN.
11. _____ Residual drug volume	K. Something that provides thrust.

CHARACTERISTICS OF THERAPEUTIC AEROSOLS

12. What influence does particle size have on aerosol therapy?

_____

13. What is the primary method of deposition for large, high-mass particles?

_____

14. Particles of 10 microns or larger tend to be deposited in what part of the respiratory tract?

What about particles between 5 and 10 microns?

A. ≥10: _____

B. 5 to 10: _____

15. In what part of the lung would you like to deposit beta-adrenergic bronchodilator medications? What particle size is needed to accomplish this goal?

A. Where: _____

B. Particle size: _____

265

Copyright © 2025, Elsevier, Inc. All rights reserved.

16. Sedimentation is an important factor in lung deposition that RTs can influence.

   A. How long is an ideal breath hold maneuver? _____

   B. How much will you increase drug deposition? _____

   C. What about drug distribution? _____

17. It is extremely difficult to predict exactly what happens to particles once they enter the lung. What is the most practical way to determine how well you are delivering a medication?

   _____

HAZARDS OF AEROSOL THERAPY

18. Nebulizers can be a source for nosocomial infections. Describe three of the CDC's recommendations for preventing this problem.

   A. _____

   B. _____

   C. _____

19. List five aerosolized substances associated with increased airway resistance.

   A. _____

   B. _____

   C. _____

   D. _____

   E. _____

20. What can you do to help prevent bronchospasm from occurring when you nebulize reactive substances?

   _____

21. Aerosolizing drugs has the potential for inducing bronchospasm. Describe four ways you can monitor this potential problem.

   A. _____

   B. _____

   C. _____

   D. _____

22. Eye irritation is most likely to occur under what circumstances?

Copyright © 2025, Elsevier, Inc. All rights reserved.

Metered Dose Inhalers

23. What is priming the MDI? When should it be done?

24. What other substances are found in MDIs that may produce clinical problems?

_____

25. What percentage of the drug in an MDI is actually deposited in the lungs? Why is there so much variability?

_____

26. List a benefit of a breath-actuated MDI.

_____

27. Put the following steps of optimal open-mouth MDI delivery in order.

   A. Hold your breath for 10 seconds.   _____

   B. Breathe out normally.   _____

   C. Wait 1 minute.   _____

   D. Actuate canister (dose).   _____

   E. Hold the MDI two fingers from mouth.   _____

   F. Slowly inhale as deeply as you can.   _____

   G. Warm and shake the canister.   _____

   H. Actuate the canister (prime).   _____

   I. Take off the cap.   _____

28. What is the difference between a spacer and a holding chamber? Does it matter?

29. Holding chambers are especially useful for what class of inhaled medications?

_____

30. How does the recommended breathing pattern with a holding chamber differ from that with a spacer or unassisted MDI?

Copyright © 2025, Elsevier, Inc. All rights reserved.

Dry Powder

31. What is a DPI? How is it powered?

32. How does DPI breathing technique differ from that recommended with an MDI?

_____

33. What patients should not use DPIs?

_____

34. In general, what is the role of the DPI in management of acute bronchospasm?

Small-Volume Nebulizers

35. List two potential power sources to drive the small-volume nebulizer.

A. _____

B. _____

36. What is the ideal flow rate and amount of solution to put in an SVN for a typical albuterol treatment?

A. Flow rate: _____

B. Amount of solution: _____

37. What is a baffle?

_____

38. What is meant by nebulizer "sputter," and why is it important to RTs?

39. What potential problem exists when you deliver an SVN via mask? How can you deal with this problem?

Copyright © 2025, Elsevier, Inc. All rights reserved.

40. Explain what is meant by the "blow-by" technique used with infants and discuss the effectiveness of this technique.

41. Explain how the Respimat soft mist inhaler works.

42. You really can't nebulize all of the solution. Explain the idea of residual volume. How broad is the range?

43. What population of pediatric patients may be considered for continuous nebulization? How is it delivered?

Small Ultrasonic Nebulizers

44. List three advantages and three disadvantages of USNs to deliver medications.

	ADVANTAGES	DISADVANTAGES
A.		
B.		
C.		

CASE STUDIES

Selection of aerosol drug delivery devices and doses.

Case 1

An alert, cooperative 52-year-old man has recently been diagnosed with chronic bronchitis. He quit smoking (60-pack-year history) 6 months ago but still has respiratory symptoms. He is in your pulmonary clinic today to receive his pulmonary function test (PFT) results and medications. The physician has ordered Atrovent and Flovent.

45. What method of delivery would you recommend for this patient?

Copyright © 2025, Elsevier, Inc. All rights reserved.

46. What other equipment is indicated?

_____

47. What general considerations for patient education would you stress for this patient?

_____

48. How will you know that he is able to perform the therapy correctly?

_____

Case 2

A 27-year-old man presents in the emergency department with acute respiratory distress. He is diagnosed with status asthmaticus. He has high-pitched diffuse wheezes, a respiratory rate of 24, heart rate of 106, and SpO_2 of 92%. His PEFR is 150 after four puffs of albuterol via MDI.

49. What are the possible options for treating this patient at this point?

_____

50. What method of bronchodilator delivery would you recommend?

_____

51. What is meant by "dose-response" assessment?

_____

Case 3

You are asked to deliver a bronchodilator to a patient in the neurologic intensive care unit. When you arrive to assess the patient, you note that she is obtunded. Breath sounds reveal scattered rhonchi and wheezing in the upper lobes.

52. What method of bronchodilator delivery would you recommend in this situation?

_____

53. What modification will you need to make?

_____

54. Because peak flow is unlikely to be performed, how will you assess the effectiveness of therapy?

_____

INTUBATED PATIENTS

55. What is the starting dose for albuterol via SVN for an intubated patient?

_____

56. What standard starting dosage is recommended for albuterol by MDI to a ventilator patient?

_____

Copyright © 2025, Elsevier, Inc. All rights reserved.

57. Where should you place the SVN in the ventilator circuit?

_____

58. When should an MDI be activated for a ventilator patient?

_____

59. What adjustments to dilution need to be made with the SVN for ventilator delivery?

_____

60. Describe the method for giving a bronchodilator to a patient on noninvasive mask ventilation.

61. Describe the method for giving a bronchodilator to a patient who is on an oscillator.

WHAT DOES THE NBRC SAY?

The following information pertains to questions 62 and 63. Circle the best answer.

Asthma has been recently diagnosed in a 16-year-old patient. The respiratory therapist is asked to teach the patient how to self-administer QVAR via MDI.

62. In addition to the inhaler, what other equipment would be needed to teach the patient?
    1. Spacer device
    2. Pulse oximeter
    3. Peak flowmeter
        A. 1 only
        B. 1 and 2 only
        C. 1 and 3 only
        D. 2 and 3 only

63. After performing the inhalation, the RT instructs the patient to perform a breath-holding maneuver. The purpose of

    this maneuver is to _____.
    A. promote a strong cough
    B. improve venous return
    C. improve inertial impaction
    D. increase medication delivery

Copyright © 2025, Elsevier, Inc. All rights reserved.   Chapter **40** **Aerosol Drug Therapy**

64. While attempting to administer albuterol via SVN to a patient who has had a recent CVA, the RT notes that the patient is unable to hold the nebulizer or keep her lips sealed on the mouthpiece. The RT should recommend

   _____.

   A. switching to an MDI
   B. utilizing an aerosol mask for delivery
   C. discontinuing the medication
   D. subcutaneous administration of the medication

65. An MDI is ordered for a patient who is intubated and being mechanically ventilated and humidified with a heat-moisture exchanger (HME). Which of the following is the most appropriate way to administer the bronchodilator?
   A. Place the MDI in the expiratory limb of the ventilator circuit.
   B. Place the MDI between the HME and the endotracheal tube.
   C. Recommend changing the delivery method to a small-volume nebulizer.
   D. Remove the HME during delivery of the drug.

66. An alert adult patient with asthma is receiving bronchodilator therapy via small volume nebulizer during a hospitalization. What recommendations should the RT make in regard to this therapy when the patient is ready for discharge?
   A. Recommend MDI instruction.
   B. Recommend oral administration of the medication.
   C. Recommend training in home use of the SVN.
   D. Recommend administration of the drug via IPPB.

67. Which of the following devices is most suitable for delivery of treprostinil?
   A. Pari LC
   B. Small particle aerosol generator
   C. A pulsed ultrasonic nebulizer
   D. Atomizer

FOOD FOR THOUGHT

68. What two inhalational drugs have proved to be an occupational risk for RTs?

   A. _____

   B. _____

69. Describe some of the physical ways to control environmental contamination when delivering medications that have potential side effects for the provider.

70. What do the terms HEPA and PAPR refer to?

   _____

Copyright © 2025, Elsevier, Inc. All rights reserved.

41 Storage and Delivery of Medical Gases

WORD WIZARD

Look up these nine terms and give a brief description.

Characteristics

1. Flammable

2. Nonflammable

3. Oxidizing

Equipment

4. Bourdon gauge

5. Thorpe tube

6. Reducing valve

7. Regulator

8. Flowmeter

9. Zone valves

CHARACTERISTICS OF MEDICAL GASES

10. List three gases that are categorized as nonflammable.

    A. _____

    B. _____

    C. _____

11. Most therapeutic gases will oxidize or support combustion. List three gases in this category.

    A. _____

    B. _____

    C. _____

12. Describe the four basic steps of the fractional distillation process.

    A. _____

    B. _____

    C. _____

    D. _____

273

Copyright © 2025, Elsevier, Inc. All rights reserved.

13. What purity level is required for medical-grade oxygen?

_____

14. Describe the two methods used to separate oxygen from air. What concentration is produced by each method?

A. _____

B. _____

15. What is the most common use of CO_2 mixtures?

_____

16. What is heliox? What is it used for in the clinical setting?

_____

17. What is the primary medical use for nitrous oxide? What are some of the hazards of nitrous oxide administration?

18. Describe two possible hazards of using nitric oxide.
    A.

    B.

19. Give the chemical symbol for each of the following medical gases.

Gas	Symbol
A. Oxygen	_____
B. Air	_____
C. Carbon dioxide	_____
D. Helium	_____
E. Nitrous oxide	_____
F. Nitric oxide	_____

Copyright © 2025, Elsevier, Inc. All rights reserved.

STORING MEDICAL GASES

20. What do the symbols * and + mean when stamped on a cylinder?

A. * _____

B. + _____

21. Identify the proper color for these gas cylinders (in the United States).

    A. Oxygen   _____

    B. Carbon dioxide   _____

    C. Nitrous oxide   _____

    D. Helium   _____

    E. Nitrogen   _____

    F. Air   _____

22. Because cylinder color is only a guideline, how do you actually determine which gas is in a tank?

_____

FILLING CYLINDERS

23. List two gases that can be stored in the liquid state at room temperature.

A. _____

B. _____

24. Explain why the pressure in a gas-filled cylinder is different from that of a liquid-filled cylinder.

25. Describe the methods for measuring the contents of a gas-filled cylinder and a liquid-filled cylinder.

A. Gas-filled:

B. Liquid-filled:

275

Copyright © 2025, Elsevier, Inc. All rights reserved.

26. What are the cylinder factors for the "E," "G," and "H" gas-filled oxygen cylinders?

E: _____

G: _____

H: _____

27. Write the formula for calculating duration of flow in minutes of gas-filled cylinders.

_____

BULK OXYGEN

28. Describe a gaseous bulk system. Be sure to discuss the manifold, the primary, and reserve banks.

29. Why do most hospitals use a liquid bulk oxygen system?

_____

30. Where are small liquid oxygen cylinders usually used?

_____

31. What is the normal working pressure for a hospital oxygen piping system?

_____

32. What are zone valves? Give two reasons you might need to use these valves.

SAFETY SYSTEMS

33. If a cylinder overheats, the pressure will rise. Describe the type of pressure release valve usually found in these cylinder stems.

Small cylinder: _____

Large cylinder: _____

34. List the three basic indexed safety systems for medical gases. Both names!

Abbreviated name	Full name
A. _____	_____
B. _____	_____
C. _____	_____

Copyright © 2025, Elsevier, Inc. All rights reserved.

35. What type of cylinder typically uses pins and holes for the safety connection system?

_____

36. What system was established to prevent accidental interchange of low-pressure medical gas connectors? What is meant by "low-pressure?"

_____

REGULATION PRESSURE AND FLOW

37. Describe the action of the following devices.

A. Reducing valve: _____

B. Flowmeter: _____

C. Regulator: _____

38. Describe the normal way each of the following is used in respiratory care.

A. Preset reducing valve:

B. Adjustable reducing valve:

C. Multiple-stage reducing valve:

39. What two hazards can be created when you open a cylinder attached to a high-pressure reducing valve?

40. What are two advantages and two disadvantages of flow restrictors?

	ADVANTAGES	DISADVANTAGES
A.		
B.		

277

Copyright © 2025, Elsevier, Inc. All rights reserved.

41. Describe the Bourdon flowmeter.

_____

42. What is the chief advantage of the Bourdon-type flowmeter?

_____

43. What do Bourdon gauges actually measure? What do Thorpe tubes measure?

  A. Bourdon: _____

  B. Thorpe: _____

44. Compare indicated flow and actual flow in a compensated Thorpe flowmeter when downstream resistance occurs.

45. What happens to the float in a compensated Thorpe tube when you connect it to a 50-psi gas source?

CASE STUDY

Case 1

A patient is to be transported from the ICU to the imaging department for a CT scan. The patient requires continuous supplemental oxygen at 10 L/min by mask. You will need to provide portable oxygen for the transport. An E cylinder is available.

46. What type of regulator is most appropriate for transport?

_____

47. How long will the cylinder last at the given flow rate if the pressure is 1000 psi?

  Formula: _____

  Calculation: _____

48. When you turn on the cylinder valve, a hissing noise is heard from the regulator. The flowmeter is off, so there must be a leak. What should you check to try to correct the leak?

  A. _____

  B. _____

Copyright © 2025, Elsevier, Inc. All rights reserved.

MEASURING CYLINDER CONTENTS

49. Calculate duration of an E cylinder with 1500 psi running at 2 L/min.

    Formula: _____

    Calculation:

    Answer: Minutes _____ Hours _____

50. Calculate the duration of an H cylinder with 1500 psi running at 2 L/min.

    Formula: _____

    Calculation:

    Answer: Minutes _____ Hours _____

WHAT DOES THE NBRC SAY?

Circle the best answer.

51. An H cylinder of oxygen is being used to deliver oxygen to a patient in a subacute care facility where no piped-in oxygen is available. The cylinder gauge shows a pressure of 1000 psi. The patient is receiving oxygen at 5 L/min by cannula. Approximately how long will the cylinder gas last at this flow rate?
    A. 1 hour
    B. 8 hours
    C. 10 hours
    D. 628 hours

52. A respiratory therapist notices that a flowmeter plugged into the wall outlet continues to read 1 L/min even though it is not turned on. What is the most appropriate action at this time?
    A. Replace the flowmeter.
    B. Include the extra liter in any calculations.
    C. Disassemble the flowmeter and replace the "O-rings."
    D. Do nothing; this is not an unusual situation.

53. A respiratory therapist has to transport a patient via air from the island of Maui to Honolulu. The patient is being manually ventilated with an oxygen flow set at 10 L/min using an E cylinder of gas. The cylinder gauge reads 2000 psi. How long will the cylinder last?
    A. 42 minutes
    B. 56 minutes
    C. 60 minutes
    D. 10 hours

Copyright © 2025, Elsevier, Inc. All rights reserved.

54. A fire breaks out in the pediatrics unit because of a faulty electrical cord. One respiratory therapist has ensured that patients with oxygen are safe. Your responsibility in this situation would be to
A. prepare to shut off the zone valves to the unit.
B. obtain an additional crash cart for emergencies.
C. obtain additional E cylinders of oxygen.
D. prepare to document the incident in the record.

FOOD FOR THOUGHT

55. Your text describes the catastrophic consequences of bulk-system failures. Describe what some of your actions might be in this type of emergency.

Copyright © 2025, Elsevier, Inc. All rights reserved.

42 Medical Gas Therapy

OXYGEN THERAPY

Let's start by reviewing the reasons for giving oxygen and how to clinically recognize those needs.

1. What is acute hypoxemia? _____

2. What are the threshold criteria for defining hypoxemia in adults according to the AARC Clinical Practice Guidelines?

   1. PaO_2 _____

   2. SaO_2 _____

3. Describe the two compensatory mechanisms of the cardiopulmonary system when faced with hypoxemia.

   A. Lungs: _____

   B. Heart: _____

4. In what acute cardiac condition is oxygen therapy especially important?

_____

5. What effect does hypoxemia have on the pulmonary blood vessels? What are the long-term consequences of this effect?

6. List three basic ways to determine when a patient needs oxygen.

   A. _____

   B. _____

   C. _____

Copyright © 2025, Elsevier, Inc. All rights reserved.

7. List six common acute clinical situations where hypoxemia is so common that oxygen therapy is usually provided.

A. _____

B. _____

C. _____

D. _____

E. _____

F. _____

8. List two signs of mild and severe hypoxia for each of the following systems.

	SYSTEM	MILD	SEVERE
A.	Respiratory		
B.	Cardiovascular		
C.	Neurologic		

PRECAUTIONS AND HAZARDS OF SUPPLEMENTAL OXYGEN THERAPY

9. Oxygen toxicity can affect what two organ systems?

A. _____

B. _____

10. The harm caused by oxygen is influenced by what two factors?

A. _____

B. _____

11. Describe the effects on the lung tissue of breathing excessive oxygen.

12. What is meant by a "vicious circle" in reference to oxygen toxicity?

Copyright © 2025, Elsevier, Inc. All rights reserved.

13. Although every patient is unique, what general rule of thumb can be applied to prevent oxygen toxicity?

14. What specific type of COPD patient is likely to experience depression of ventilatory drive while breathing oxygen?

_____

15. When should oxygen be withheld from a hypoxic COPD patient to avoid depressing ventilation?

_____

16. During what time period after birth is a preemie likely to develop ROP?

_____

17. How can you reduce the risk of ROP?

_____

18. Describe how oxygen can cause atelectasis.

19. How can you reduce the risk of absorption atelectasis?

_____

20. What is the fire triangle?

21. What is the biggest hazard in the home setting?

Copyright © 2025, Elsevier, Inc. All rights reserved.

22. The three basic categories of oxygen delivery systems are low flow, high flow, and reservoir. Match the category to the description below.

	CATEGORY	DESCRIPTION
A.	Low flow	1. Always exceeds patient's inspiratory needs
B.	Reservoir	2. Provides some of patient's inspiratory needs
C.	High flow	3. May meet needs if no leaks occur

LOW FLOW

23. When should you attach the cannula to a bubble humidifier?

_____

24. What maximum flow does the text suggest for newborns?

_____

25. How does the patient's breathing pattern affect the F_IO_2 delivered to the lungs when using a low-flow device such as a cannula?

26. What is the primary disadvantage of the transtracheal catheter?

27. What range of F_IO_2 is usually delivered by low-flow devices?

_____

28. Because you can't tell exactly how much oxygen the patient is receiving at any given moment from a cannula or any low-flow device, how can you assess the effects of administering the drug?

_____

29. In what setting are reservoir cannulas usually used?

_____

Copyright © 2025, Elsevier, Inc. All rights reserved.

30. Fill in the information about oxygen masks.

	MASK	F_IO_2 RANGE	ADVANTAGE	DISADVANTAGE
A.	Simple			
B.	Partial rebreathing			
C.	Nonrebreathing			

31. What is the primary difference between the partial rebreathing and nonrebreathing masks?

_____

32. How can you tell if a nonrebreathing mask has an adequate flow rate?

_____

33. Give a solution for each of these common problems with reservoir masks.

Problem	Solution
A. No gas felt from cannula	_____
B. Humidifier pop-off activated	_____
C. Mask causes claustrophobia	_____
D. Bag collapses on inspiration	_____
E. Bag fully inflated on inspiration	_____

34. Describe the effects of varying the jet size or entrainment port opening on F_IO_2 and total flow rate.

	FACTOR	INCREASED SIZE	DECREASED SIZE
A.	Jet 1. F_IO_2 2. Flow		
B.	Port 1. F_IO_2 2. Flow		

Copyright © 2025, Elsevier, Inc. All rights reserved.

35. Fill in the air-to-oxygen ratios for the following oxygen concentrations.

A. 100% _____

B. 60% _____

C. 40% _____

D. 35% _____

E. 30% _____

F. 24% _____

36. Why does the AEM have larger openings on the side of the mask than a simple oxygen mask?

_____

37. What effect does raising the delivered flow from the flowmeter have on the F_IO_2 delivered by an AEM?

_____

38. How do you boost the total flow when using an AEM?

_____

39. There are four devices used to deliver gas from an air-entrainment nebulizer to the patient. Choose the device(s) that fits each of the following patients. (See Figure 38-16 in your text.)

Patient	Aerosol Delivery Device
A. Tracheostomy tube	_____
B. Endotracheal tube	_____
C. Intact upper airway	_____
D. After nasal surgery	_____

40. Describe an easy way to tell if an air-entrainment nebulizer is providing sufficient gas to meet the patient's needs.

41. Give one example of a specialized flow generator that produces an aerosol.

_____

42. What effect does downstream resistance to flow have on F_IO_2 and total flow delivered by a typical AEM or nebulizer entrainment system?

Copyright © 2025, Elsevier, Inc. All rights reserved.

43. What is the oxygen–to-air entrainment ratio and total flow for a patient who is receiving 60% oxygen via an entrainment nebulizer with the flowmeter set at 10 L/min?

    A. Step 1: Compute the ratio.

        Formula: _____

        Calculation: _____

        Reduce answer to get ratio: _____

    B. Step 2: Add the parts.

    C. Step 3: Multiply the sum of the parts by the O_2 flow rate.

HIGH-FLOW SYSTEMS AND HYPOXEMIA

High-flow oxygen systems are a valuable new tool for managing serious hypoxemia.

44. What three main features make the Vapotherm and the Fisher and Paykel's Optiflow high-flow systems useful for treating moderate hypoxemia?

45. What are the major limitations of these devices?

46. What device could you use during resuscitation or in the emergency setting to administer 100% oxygen?

Copyright © 2025, Elsevier, Inc. All rights reserved.

47. Compare the monoplace and multiplace hyperbaric chambers.

	CHAMBER	O$_2$ DELIVERY	PATIENT	STAFF
A.	Monoplace			
B.	Multiplace			

48. List three acute and three chronic conditions in which HBO is indicated.

Acute   **Chronic**

A. _____   _____

B. _____   _____

C. _____   _____

49. Under what circumstances is HBO indicated in cases of carbon monoxide poisoning?

OTHER GASES

50. Two other therapeutic gases are commonly administered by RTs. Give indications for each.

Gas   **Indications**

A. NO   _____

            _____

B. Helium   _____

            _____

51. What other gas is always mixed with helium? What is the most common combination?

_____

52. What physical property of helium results in decreased work of breathing?

_____

Copyright © 2025, Elsevier, Inc. All rights reserved.

Case 1

A 52-year-old college professor is admitted for chest pain and possible myocardial infarction (MI). Electrocardiogram (ECG) monitoring reveals sinus tachycardia. The chest pain has been decreased by the administration of nitroglycerin. Respirations are 20 per minute, and SpO_2 on room air is 92%.

53. What is your assessment of this patient's oxygenation status?

54. What is your recommendation in regard to administration of supplemental oxygen?

Case 2

A man has been admitted for exacerbation of his COPD. The patient is receiving oxygen at 2 L/min via nasal cannula. The pulse oximeter shows a saturation of 94% while at rest. The nurse calls you to ask for your assistance in evaluation of the patient's dyspnea during ambulation.

55. What changes occur in a breathing pattern during exercise?

_____

56. How are low-flow oxygen devices affected by changes in a breathing pattern?

_____

57. How would you assess dyspnea on ambulation for a patient wearing oxygen?

Case 3

A patient is recovering from surgery following a head injury. The patient is trached and requires supplemental oxygen at 60% via T-piece. The flowmeter is set at 12 L/min. Each time the patient inhales, the mist exiting the T-piece disappears.

58. Air-entrainment nebulizers are considered high-flow delivery systems. Discuss this in terms of the disappearing mist.

_____

59. What should be added to the T-piece to help deal with this problem?

_____

60. Describe a common method of increasing the delivered flow when administering high F_IO_2 via air-entrainment nebulizers. _____

289

Copyright © 2025, Elsevier, Inc. All rights reserved.

61. What is the oxygen-to-air entrainment ratio for 60%?

_____

62. What is the total flow in the system described in this case?

_____

WHAT DOES THE NBRC SAY?

Circle the best answer.

63. During a suctioning procedure a patient experiences tachycardia with PVCs. Which of the following could be responsible for this response?
    A. Inadequate vacuum pressure.
    B. Lack of sterile technique during the procedure.
    C. Fear of the suctioning procedure.
    D. Inadequate preoxygenation.

64. A patient with a history of carbon dioxide retention is receiving oxygen at 6 L/min via nasal cannula. He is becoming lethargic and difficult to arouse. In regard to the oxygen delivery, what change would you recommend?
    A. Change to a 40% Venturi mask.
    B. Maintain the present therapy.
    C. Change to a partial rebreathing mask.
    D. Reduce the flow to 2 L/min and obtain an ABG.

65. A newborn requires oxygen therapy. Which of the following methods of delivery would you select?
    A. Partial rebreathing mask
    B. Oxygen hood
    C. Venturi mask
    D. Oxygen tent

66. A patient is receiving oxygen therapy from a nonrebreathing mask with a flow rate of 10 L/min. The respiratory therapist observes the bag deflating with each inspiration. What action is indicated in this situation?
    A. Replace the mask with a cannula.
    B. Immediately perform pulse oximetry.
    C. Increase the flow to the mask.
    D. Change to a Venturi mask.

67. A patient is to receive a mixture of helium and oxygen. Which of the following delivery devices would be appropriate?
    A. Nasal cannula
    B. Oxygen tent
    C. Venturi mask
    D. Nonrebreathing mask

68. An 80/20 mixture of helium and oxygen is administered. An oxygen flowmeter is set at 10 L/min. What is the actual flow delivered to the patient?
    A. 10 L
    B. 14 L
    C. 16 L
    D. 18 L

69. A patient is receiving 40% oxygen via an air-entrainment mask with the flowmeter set at 8 L/min. What is the total flow delivered to the patient?
    A. 24 L/min
    B. 32 L/min
    C. 40 L/min
    D. 48 L/min

290

Copyright © 2025, Elsevier, Inc. All rights reserved.

70. A patient requires a flow rate of 40 L/min to meet his inspiratory demand for gas. He is to receive oxygen via a Venturi mask set at 24%. What is the minimum setting on the flowmeter to produce the appropriate flow?
A. 1 L/min
B. 2 L/min
C. 3 L/min
D. 4 L/min

71. Which of the following should be used to deliver a 70:30 heliox mixture?
A. Nonrebreathing mask
B. Simple mask
C. Aerosol mask
D. Endotracheal tube

FOOD FOR THOUGHT

72. Why does common use of the term "100% nonrebreather" create a clinical problem?

73. Why would an AEM be preferred over an air-entrainment nebulizer for a patient who has asthma or COPD?

74. Why is protocol-based oxygen therapy beneficial? What should well-designed protocols include?

75. Following delivery of a 70:30 heliox mixture to a patient she complains of difficulty coughing. What should you do?

Copyright © 2025, Elsevier, Inc. All rights reserved.

43 Lung Expansion Therapy

WORD WIZARD

For each of the following terms or treatments, give a simple, short explanation in lay terms that your patient could understand.

1. Atelectasis: "When you don't take deep breaths…"

   _____

2. Incentive spirometer (IS):

   A. "The purpose of this treatment is to…"

      _____

   B. "This device will…" _____

3. Sustained maximal inspiration (SMI): "I want you to take…"

   _____

4. Continuous positive airway pressure (CPAP)

   A. "This treatment will…" _____

   B. "I am going to put a mask on your face…"

      _____

MEET THE OBJECTIVES

Answer the following questions to test your understanding of this chapter's objectives.

5. What is the definition of atelectasis?

   _____

6. What is resorption atelectasis, and when is it likely to occur?

7. What causes compression atelectasis?

Copyright © 2025, Elsevier, Inc. All rights reserved.

8. Why are postoperative patients at highest risk for development of atelectasis?

9. Which specific group of postoperative patients is at highest risk of developing atelectasis?
_____

10. List two other types of patients who have increased likelihood of developing atelectasis. Explain why.
   A. _____
   B. _____

11. Explain how each of the following may help provide clues that atelectasis is present or likely.
   A. History

   B. Breath sounds

   C. Respiratory rate

   D. Heart rate

   E. Chest radiography

Copyright © 2025, Elsevier, Inc. All rights reserved.

12. List indications, contraindications, and hazards of incentive spirometry.
    A. Indications

        1. _____

        2. _____

        3. _____

    B. Contraindications

        1. _____

        2. _____

        3. _____

    C. Hazards

        1. _____

        2. _____

13. Consider the complication of hyperventilation and pain. What are your ideas about dealing with these problems?
    A. Hyperventilation:

    B. Pain:

14. List three current positive airway pressure (PAP) therapies.

    A. _____

    B. _____

    C. _____

15. List four factors that contribute to the benefit of PEP, flutter, and CPAP.

    A. _____

    B. _____

    C. _____

    D. _____

16. List two contraindications to CPAP therapy.

    A. _____

    B. _____

Copyright © 2025, Elsevier, Inc. All rights reserved.

17. What alarm system is essential for monitoring patients receiving continuous mask CPAP?

18. List three complications of prolonged bed rest. How would you remedy this problem?

    A.

    B.

    C.

    Remedy:

SUMMARY CHECKLIST

Complete the following sentences by writing a brief response in the spaces provided.

19. What causes atelectasis?

20. Describe a patient population that is at risk of atelectasis.

21. What part of a patient's history puts them at an additional risk for atelectasis?

22. How is the presence of atelectasis sometimes confirmed?

23. What breathing pattern do patients with atelectasis usually demonstrate?

24. What is the most common blood gas problem associated with lung expansion therapy?

Copyright © 2025, Elsevier, Inc. All rights reserved.

Case 1

An alert 34-year-old man is admitted for a hernia repair. He smokes two packs of cigarettes per day. Following surgery, the physician asks for your recommendation for therapy to prevent lung complications. The patient's vital capacity is 1.4 L and he weighs 80 kg, his predicted body weight. He complains of cough but produces no sputum.

25. Discuss potential risk factors for atelectasis in this case.

_____

26. What therapy would you recommend for prevention of atelectasis for this patient?

_____

Case 2

A 70-year-old, 5-foot 2-inch female patient is immobilized following hip replacement. Her predicted inspiratory capacity is 1.8 L. She is performing incentive spirometry at 500 ml per breath. Breath sounds reveal bilateral basilar crackles, and she is coughing up lots of thick mucus.

27. What is the minimum acceptable volume for incentive spirometry for this patient according to her predicted IC and her measured volume?

_____

28. What treatment would you recommend adding to the therapeutic regimen at this time?

_____

WHAT DOES THE NBRC SAY?

Circle the best answer.

29. A patient complains of a "tingling" feeling in her lips during an incentive spirometry treatment. The RT should

    instruct the patient to _____.
    A. breathe more slowly
    B. take smaller breaths
    C. continue with the treatment as ordered
    D. exhale through pursed lips after each breath

30. Which of the following alarms is a vital part of the system when setting up CPAP therapy for treatment of atelectasis?
    A. Exhaled volume
    B. High respiratory rate
    C. Pulse oximetry
    D. Low pressure

31. During administration of IPPB therapy, the practitioner observes the system pressure rise suddenly at the end of

    inspiration. The RT should instruct the patient to _____.
    A. "Help the machine give you a deep breath"
    B. "Inhale slowly along with the machine"
    C. "Exhale gently and normally"
    D. "Exhale through pursed lips after each breath"

Copyright © 2025, Elsevier, Inc. All rights reserved.

32. A patient is having difficulty initiating each breath with an IPPB machine. The practitioner should adjust the

    _____.
    A. pressure limit
    B. peak flow
    C. F_IO_2
    D. sensitivity

33. Which control is used to increase the volume delivered by an IPPB machine?
    A. Pressure limit
    B. Peak flow
    C. F_IO_2
    D. Sensitivity

34. Continuous positive airway pressure is used to increase which of the following?
    A. Functional residual capacity
    B. Peak expiratory flow rate
    C. FEV_1
    D. Arterial carbon dioxide levels

35. An IPPB machine cycles on with the patient effort but does not shut off. The most likely cause of this problem is

    _____.
    A. the pressure is set too low
    B. the sensitivity is set incorrectly
    C. there is a leak in the system
    D. the patient is not blowing out hard enough

36. How should you instruct a patient to breathe during incentive spirometry?
    A. "Exhale gently, then inhale rapidly through the spirometer."
    B. "Inhale deeply and rapidly through the spirometer."
    C. "Exhale until your lungs are empty, then inhale and hold your breath."
    D. "Exhale normally, then inhale slowly and deeply and hold your breath."

37. How often should a patient be instructed to use the incentive spirometer after being taught to perform the procedure correctly?
    A. 10 breaths, four times per day
    B. 6 to 10 breaths every hour
    C. 10 to 20 breaths every 2 hours
    D. 6 to 8 breaths three times daily

38. A patient who has had surgery for an abdominal aortic aneurysm suffers from arrhythmias and hypotension after surgery. The physician asks for your recommendation for lung expansion therapy. The best choice in this situation

    would be _____.
    A. IS
    B. IPPB
    C. PEP
    D. CPAP

39. When adjusting the flow rate control on an IPPB machine, the RT would be altering the _____.
    A. maximum pressure delivered by the device
    B. effort required to initiate a breath
    C. volume delivered by the machine
    D. inspiratory time for a given breath

FOOD FOR THOUGHT

40. A really interesting topic in critical care is how best to reinflate the acutely restricted or atelectatic lung. "Lung recruitment maneuvers" is the correct name. Search for this term and explain briefly, in your own words, how a lung recruitment maneuver is done.

297

Copyright © 2025, Elsevier, Inc. All rights reserved.

44 Airway Clearance Therapy

WORD WIZARD

Write out each of these acronyms.

1. ACBT _____

2. PEP _____

3. AD _____

4. PDPV _____

5. CPT _____

6. CPAP _____

7. EPAP _____

8. FET _____

9. HFCWC _____

10. HZ _____

11. ICP _____

12. IPV _____

13. MI-E _____

AIRWAY CLEARANCE

14. List the four phases of the normal cough. Give examples of impairments for each.

Phase	Impairments
A. _____	_____
B. _____	_____
C. _____	_____
D. _____	_____

15. Compare the effects of full and partial airway obstruction caused by retained secretions.

   A. Full obstruction, or _____ plugging, results in _____.

   B. Partial obstruction increases _____ of breathing and leads to air _____.

Copyright © 2025, Elsevier, Inc. All rights reserved.

16. List three conditions that may cause internal obstruction or external compression of the airway lumen (opening).

    A. _____

    B. _____

    C. _____

17. List two obstructive lung diseases that result in excessive secretion of mucus and impairment of normal clearance.

    A. _____

    B. _____

18. List four neurologic or musculoskeletal conditions that impair cough.

    A. _____

    B. _____

    C. _____

    D. _____

SECRETION MANAGEMENT: GOALS AND INDICATIONS

19. List four acute conditions in which bronchial hygiene is indicated.

    A. _____

    B. _____

    C. _____

    D. _____

20. Discuss bronchial hygiene therapy for chronic lung conditions. How much sputum needs to be produced daily for the therapy to be useful? What are three typical diseases that we treat?

21. Describe the two well-documented preventive, or prophylactic, uses of bronchial hygiene therapy.
    A.

    B.

299

Copyright © 2025, Elsevier, Inc. All rights reserved.

22. Give a brief explanation of the significance of each factor listed below.

Factor	Significance
A. History	_____
B. Airway	_____
C. Chest radiograph	_____
D. Breath sounds	_____
E. Vital signs	_____

BRONCHIAL HYGIENE METHODS

23. Postural drainage therapy includes up to four components, not counting cough. What are they?

A. _____

B. _____

C. _____

D. _____

24. List two absolute and two relative contraindications to turning.
A. Absolute

1. _____

2. _____

B. Relative

1. _____

2. _____

25. How long should you wait to schedule postural drainage after a patient eats? Why?

_____

26. What is the minimum range of time for effective application of postural drainage therapy?

_____

27. Give a recommended intervention for each of the complications of postural drainage listed below.

Complication	Interventions
A. Hypoxemia	_____
B. Increased ICP	_____
C. Acute hypotension	_____
D. Pulmonary bleeding	_____
E. Vomiting	_____
F. Bronchospasm	_____
G. Cardiac dysrhythmias	_____

Copyright © 2025, Elsevier, Inc. All rights reserved.

28. How long does it take to determine the effectiveness of postural drainage? If therapy is effective, how often should you reevaluate in the hospital? In the home?

   A. How long? _____

   B. Reevaluate hospital patients? _____

   C. Reevaluate home patients? _____

29. List five factors that must be documented after each postural drainage treatment:

   A. _____

   B. _____

   C. _____

   D. _____

   E. _____

30. Describe percussion and vibration as techniques to loosen secretions. Are they really effective?

31. Compare manual and mechanical methods of percussion and vibration.

Coughing and Related Expulsion Techniques
32. How would you position a patient (ideally) for an effective cough?

33. Standard directed cough must frequently be modified. Give three examples of types of patients who may need modified cough techniques.

   A. _____

   B. _____

   C. _____

34. What is splinting? _____

35. What special form of cough assistance is used with patients who have neuromuscular conditions?

   _____

Copyright © 2025, Elsevier, Inc. All rights reserved.

36. Describe the forced expiratory technique (FET).

37. Describe the three repeated cycles of the ACB technique.

 A. _____

 B. _____

 C. _____

38. What is the primary problem with autogenic drainage?

 _____

39. Describe the two cycles of MI-E in terms of time and pressure.
 A. Inspiratory:

 B. Expiratory:

Positive Airway Pressure

40. Positive airway pressure is a popular way to help mobilize secretions. What are the four indications for PAP adjuncts according to the AARC Clinical Practice Guidelines?

 A. _____

 B. _____

 C. _____

 D. _____

41. What type of monitoring is essential regardless of the equipment used to deliver positive airway pressure to help mobilize secretions?

Copyright © 2025, Elsevier, Inc. All rights reserved.

High-Frequency Compression/Oscillation of the Chest Wall

42. Describe the two general approaches to oscillation.

    A. _____

    B. _____

43. Describe the way IPV delivers gas to the airway.

44. Describe four of the benefits or advantages of the flutter valve as a secretion management tool.

    A. _____

    B. _____

    C. _____

    D. _____

Mobilization and Exercise

45. Describe the benefits of adding exercise as a mobilization technique.

46. What should you specifically monitor when exercising patients with lung problems?

CASE STUDIES

Case 1

A 60-year-old professor who has had a colon resection for an intestinal tumor is receiving incentive spirometry to help expand his lungs. You are asked to assess the patient for retained secretions. Auscultation reveals coarse rhonchi bilaterally in the upper lobes. A few scattered crackles are heard in the bases. SpO_2 on room air is 94%. The patient states he is unable to cough up anything "because it hurts too much."

47. What technique could you use to decrease the pain associated with cough in a postoperative patient?

    _____

48. What type of cough would you teach him?

    _____

Copyright © 2025, Elsevier, Inc. All rights reserved.

A 75-year-old woman with bronchiectasis states she coughs up "cups of awful mucus every day." She is admitted with a diagnosis of pneumonia.

49. What therapy is indicated while this patient is in the hospital?

_____

As you provide the therapy, you find out that the patient is a widow who lives alone. She takes albuterol treatments via SVN when she has difficulty breathing.

50. What therapy alternatives could you recommend for home use?

_____

WHAT DOES THE NBRC SAY?

Circle the best answer.

51. During the initial treatment, a PEP device is set to deliver a pressure of 15 cm H_2O. The patient complains of dyspnea and can maintain exhalation only for a short period of time. Which of the following should the RT recommend?
    A. Decrease the PEP level to 10 cm H_2O.
    B. Increase the PEP level to 20 cm H_2O.
    C. Discontinue the PEP therapy.
    D. Add a bronchodilator to the PEP therapy.

52. A patient is lying on her left side, turned one-quarter toward her back, with the head of the bed down. What division of the lung is being drained?
    A. Lateral segments of the right lower lobe
    B. Right middle lobe
    C. Left upper lobe, lingular segments
    D. Posterior segment of the right upper lobe

53. A patient is receiving postural drainage in the Trendelenburg position. The patient begins to cough uncontrollably. What action should the RT take at this time?
    A. Encourage the patient to use a huff cough.
    B. Administer oxygen therapy.
    C. Administer a bronchodilator.
    D. Raise the head of the bed.

54. A COPD patient with left lower lobe infiltrates is unable to tolerate a head-down position for postural drainage. What action would you recommend?
    A. Perform the drainage with the head of the bed raised.
    B. Do not perform the therapy until 2 hours after the last meal.
    C. Administer a bronchodilator prior to the postural drainage.
    D. Notify the physician and suggest a different secretion management technique.

55. Active patient participation is an important part of which of the following procedures?
    1. Postural drainage
    2. Directed cough techniques
    3. Airway suctioning
    4. Positive expiratory pressure (PEP)

    A. 1 and 2
    B. 2 and 4
    C. 1 and 3
    D. 3 and 4

Copyright © 2025, Elsevier, Inc. All rights reserved.

56. An RT is preparing a patient with bronchiectasis for discharge. Which of the following techniques would be most appropriate for self-administered therapy in the home?
    A. IPPB
    B. Flutter
    C. Suctioning
    D. Percussion and postural drainage

FOOD FOR THOUGHT

57. How does hydration affect secretion clearance? What respiratory therapy modality can augment hydration of the airway?

58. What are the settings for a patient using the MIE device? What added feature do the newer MIE devices incorporate?

Copyright © 2025, Elsevier, Inc. All rights reserved.

45 Respiratory Failure and the Need for Ventilatory Support

WORD WIZARD

Match the definitions to these seven concepts.

_____ Auto-PEEP

_____ Barotrauma

_____ Dynamic hyperinflation

_____ Type I respiratory failure

_____ Type II respiratory failure

_____ Respiratory alternans

_____ Pressure-time index

_____ Work of breathing

A. Switching from abdominal to ribcage breathing.
B. Another term for dynamic hyperinflation
C. The oxygen is too low.
D. The carbon dioxide is too high.
E. The physiologic cost of increased dead space and resistance.
F. Hyperinflation, elevated airway pressures, and procedures lead to this harmful outcome.
G. Low rates, high flows, and moderate volumes avoid this harmful outcome.
H. Endurance depends on magnitude of respiratory load and strength and duration of effort

RESPIRATORY FAILURE

1. Complete this sentence: "Put simply, respiratory failure is the _____."

2. Define the blood gas criteria for respiratory failure.

   A. PaO_2: _____

   B. $PaCO_2$: _____

3. What are the two general types of respiratory failure based on the type of physiologic impairment?

   A. Type I: _____

   B. Type II: _____

4. Give and example of an arterial blood gas presentation of acute hypoxemic respiratory failure due to $\dot{V}/\dot{Q}$ mismatch or shunt?

   _____

5. What is the relationship between $PaCO_2$ and alveolar ventilation?

307

Copyright © 2025, Elsevier, Inc. All rights reserved.

6. Give two examples of specific disorders responsible for acute hypercapnic respiratory failure (Type II).

    A. Decreased ventilatory drive

        1. _____

        2. _____

    B. Respiratory muscle fatigue/failure

        1. _____

        2. _____

    C. Increased work of breathing

        1. _____

        2. _____

7. Give an example of a condition that could cause greatly increased CO_2 production.

_____

ACUTE-ON-CHRONIC RESPIRATORY FAILURE

8. How does the body compensate for chronically elevated carbon dioxide levels associated with COPD or obesity hypoventilation syndrome? _____

9. Describe what happens to the normal blood gas classification of respiratory failure in patients with chronic respiratory failure.

10. Identify five of the most common precipitating factors that lead to acute-on-chronic failure.

    A. _____

    B. _____

    C. _____

    D. _____

    E. _____

11. List four treatment goals for this group of patients.

    A. _____

    B. _____

    C. _____

    D. _____

Copyright © 2025, Elsevier, Inc. All rights reserved.

12. Identify the likely causes of pulmonary complications from treating acute respiratory failure.

    A. Emboli _____

    B. Barotrauma _____

    C. Infection _____

13. Give one example of each of these nonpulmonary complications that can happen to a patient in the ICU.

    A. Cardiac _____

    B. Gastrointestinal _____

    C. Renal _____

INDICATIONS FOR VENTILATORY SUPPORT

14. What is the goal of mechanical ventilation?

_____

15. Fill in the following table regarding the physiologic indicators for ventilatory support.

Mechanism	Normal and Critical Values
A. $PaCO_2$	_____
B. pH	_____
C. VC (ml/kg)	_____
D. MIP	_____
E. MVV	_____
F. V_E	_____
G. V_D/V_T	_____
H. $P(A - a)O_2$ on 100%	_____
I. P/F ratio	_____

16. What P/F ratio is considered an indicator of profoundly impaired oxygenation?

17. Why is it useful to consider pH when evaluating carbon dioxide levels to determine the need to intubate and ventilate a patient?

_____

Copyright © 2025, Elsevier, Inc. All rights reserved.

18. Define "MIP" and give the minimal value for most patients.

    A. _____

    B. _____

19. What patient group is most likely to develop respiratory muscle weakness?

    _____

20. List three conditions that frequently lead to respiratory muscle fatigue.

    A. _____

    B. _____

    C. _____

STRATEGIES

21. Define noninvasive ventilation.

22. NIV can blow off the CO_2 and improve the hypoxemia via several mechanisms. List three of them.

    A. _____

    B. _____

    C. _____

23. NIV is useful for treating COPD with respiratory failure. State two benefits of this therapy.

    A. When is NIV useful for COPD?

    B. When is it less effective?

    C. Do COPD patients actually tolerate this procedure?

Copyright © 2025, Elsevier, Inc. All rights reserved.

24. What cardiac condition is also treated by NIV?

25. Is NIV useful for treating ARDS? What does the evidence show?

26. Why is NIV unlikely to help with obesity hypoventilation syndrome?

INVASIVE VENTILATORY SUPPORT

27. List the three variables you will set in volume ventilation.

A. _____

B. _____

C. _____

28. Name the three set variables in pressure ventilation.

A. _____

B. _____

C. _____

29. What two variables are always set by the operator regardless of volume or pressure modes?

A. _____

B. _____

SPECIAL CASES

30. What is the main strategy for reducing lung injury in ARDS?

31. How does hyperventilation result in reduced ICP in head injury? What is the target $PaCO_2$ in these cases?

_____

Copyright © 2025, Elsevier, Inc. All rights reserved.

32. What is the chief concern regarding use of PEEP to increase oxygenation in patients with acute head injuries?

33. Air-trapping, or hyperinflation, as a result of obstructive lung disease causes what two complications in mechanically ventilated patients?

    A. _____

    B. _____

34. How is tidal volume and flow rate manipulated to reduce complications in mechanically ventilated COPD patients?

    A. Tidal volume _____

    B. Flow rate _____

35. What surprising technique was found to reduce auto-PEEP?

    _____

36. What is the specific goal in regard to CO_2 in respiratory failure in the chronic hypercapnic patient with COPD?

SUMMARY CHECKLIST

Complete the following by writing a brief answer in the spaces provided.

37. What carbon dioxide and oxygen levels are used to identify acute respiratory failure?

38. What are some causes of hypoxemic respiratory failure?

39. How is chronic respiratory failure represented in ABGs?

40. What is the most common cause of respiratory muscle fatigue?

Copyright © 2025, Elsevier, Inc. All rights reserved.

41. What type of patients should undergo noninvasive ventilation in the acute setting?

42. What is the goal of therapy in acute hypercapnic respiratory failure?

CASE STUDIES

Case 1

An alert, anxious 25-year-old woman presents in the emergency department complaining of chills, fever, and shortness of breath. An arterial blood gas is drawn on room air with these results:

pH	7.45
$PaCO_2$	32 mm Hg
PaO_2	50 mm Hg
HCO_3^-	23 mEq/L

43. Interpret this blood gas. _____

44. What is the A-a gradient? _____

45. What type of respiratory failure is present? _____

46. What do you recommend for initial respiratory treatment?

Case 2

A 27-year-old is brought to the emergency department by paramedics following a drug overdose. The patient is obtunded. Blood gases are drawn on room air:

pH	7.24
$PaCO_2$	60 mm Hg
PaO_2	65 mm Hg
HCO_3^-	26 mEq/L

47. Interpret this blood gas. _____

48. What is the A-a gradient? _____

49. What type of respiratory failure is present? _____

50. What is the appropriate initial respiratory treatment in this case?

Copyright © 2025, Elsevier, Inc. All rights reserved.

An alert 56-year-old man with a history of COPD presents in the emergency department complaining of dyspnea, which has worsened over the last few days. A blood gas is drawn on room air:

pH	7.26
$PaCO_2$	70 mm Hg
PaO_2	50 mm Hg
HCO_3^-	32 mEq/L

51. Interpret this blood gas. _____

52. What is the A-a gradient? _____

53. What type of respiratory failure is present? _____

54. What initial respiratory treatments are indicated? What are we trying to avoid?

WHAT DOES THE NBRC SAY?

Circle the best answer.

55. An RT is asked to evaluate a lethargic 50-year-old woman who is in respiratory distress following abdominal surgery. She is breathing spontaneously on a 50% air-entrainment mask at 32 breaths per minute. ABG results show:

pH	7.28
$PaCO_2$	55 mm Hg
PaO_2	60 mm Hg
HCO_3^-	26 mEq/L

Based on this information, what would you recommend?
A. Provide intubation and mechanical ventilation.
B. Increase the F_IO_2 to 1.0.
C. Administer CPAP.
D. Administer bronchodilator therapy via SVN.

56. An alert, anxious 60-year-old man with a history of CHF presents in the ED with respiratory distress. Auscultation reveals bilateral inspiratory crackles. He has peripheral edema. ABG results drawn on a partial rebreathing mask show:

pH	7.45
$PaCO_2$	35 mm Hg
PaO_2	40 mm Hg
HCO_3^-	23 mEq/L

The most appropriate therapy for improving oxygenation would be to
A. provide intubation and mechanical ventilation.
B. administer oxygen therapy via nonrebreathing mask.
C. administer oxygen therapy via CPAP.
D. administer bronchodilator therapy via SVN.

Copyright © 2025, Elsevier, Inc. All rights reserved.

57. An adult patient is being mechanically ventilated following respiratory failure. Settings are:

Tidal volume	600 ml
Rate	12
Mode	AC/VC
F_IO_2	0.60
PEEP	3 cm H_2O

ABGs show

pH	7.37
$PaCO_2$	41 mm Hg
PaO_2	43 mm Hg
HCO_3^-	22 mEq/L

Which of the following ventilator changes would you recommend at this time?
A. Increase the F_IO_2.
B. Decrease the volume.
C. Increase the rate.
D. Increase the PEEP.

58. A patient with a history of hypercapnia and COPD is intubated and placed on the ventilator following respiratory failure. 24 hours later, the patient is alert and breathing spontaneously.

Settings are

Tidal volume	650 ml
Rate	12
Mode	AC/VC
F_IO_2	0.30
PEEP	0 cm H_2O

ABGs show:

pH	7.48
$PaCO_2$	41 mm Hg
PaO_2	60 mm Hg
HCO_3^-	30 mEq/L

Which of the following ventilator changes would you recommend at this time?
A. Decrease the F_IO_2.
B. Decrease the volume.
C. Change to pressure-controlled ventilation (PCV).
D. Change to continuous positive airway pressure (CPAP).

59. A 77-year-old man with COPD is admitted with acute bronchitis. Room air blood gas results show

pH	7.52
$PaCO_2$	45 mm Hg
PaO_2	50 mm Hg
HCO_3^-	36 mEq/L

What intervention would be appropriate at this time?
A. CPAP with 24% oxygen
B. 28% Air entrainment mask
C. Nasal cannula at 5 L/min
D. Simple mask at 8 L/min

FOOD FOR THOUGHT

60. What clinical situations or conditions suggest using ABGs to evaluate the need to intubate and ventilate? Compare this with situations better assessed by measures such as VC and MIP.

315

Copyright © 2025, Elsevier, Inc. All rights reserved.

46 Mechanical Ventilators

WORD WIZARD

Match these definitions to the key terms.

Definitions	Terms
1. _____ Breath initiated by the ventilator.	A. Spontaneous breath
2. _____ Causes a breath to end.	B. Control variable
3. _____ Manipulated by machine to cause inspiration.	C. Limit variable
4. _____ Controls the magnitude of inspiration.	D. Cycle variable
5. _____ Combination of machine and spontaneous breaths.	E. Intermittent mandatory ventilation
6. _____ Machine breaths only—no spontaneous breaths.	F. Trigger variable
7. _____ Spontaneous breaths only—no machine breaths.	G. CMV
8. _____ Causes a breath to begin.	H. CSV
9. _____ Breath initiated and ended by the patient.	I. Mandatory breath

HOW VENTILATORS WORK

10. What is a ventilator?

11. Describe the desired output of the ventilator in terms of the patient.

   _____

12. Identify two settings where ventilators can use rechargeable battery power sources.

   A. _____

   B. _____

13. How are most modern intensive care ventilators powered?

   _____

Copyright © 2025, Elsevier, Inc. All rights reserved.

14. What does the output control valve do?

    A. Regulates: _____

    B. Shapes: _____

15. How do electrical circuits control ventilator operations?

VENTILATOR DISPLAYS AND ALARM SETTINGS

16. List four ways monitored data can be displayed. Give an example of each.

    A. _____

    B. _____

    C. _____

    D. _____

17. What is the purpose of a ventilator alarm?

18. What is an event? Explain the levels of priority with an example of each.
    Event:

    Level 1: _____

    Level 2: _____

    Level 3: _____

    Level 4: _____

19. How do ventilators display alarms? Does this present any problems?

20. What two factors can cause pressure, volume, and flow to differ from the set values to the output values?

    A. _____

    B. _____

IDENTIFYING MODES OF MECHANICAL VENTILATION

21. Define the phrase "mode of ventilation" in your own words.

_____

Copyright © 2025, Elsevier, Inc. All rights reserved.

22. List the 10 maxims for understanding modes as described in this chapter.

    1. _____

    2. _____

    3. _____

    4. _____

    5. _____

    6. _____

    7. _____

    8. _____

    9. _____

    10. _____

23. What is inspiratory time? What does it equal?

24. What is expiratory time?

25. Define *work* as it relates to a patient's *work* of breathing.

26. How is a pressure support breath cycled?

27. Define patient triggering.

28. Define machine triggering.

29. Define patient cycling.

30. Define machine cycling.

Copyright © 2025, Elsevier, Inc. All rights reserved.

31. List the three basic breath sequences and briefly describe each.

A. _____

B. _____

C. _____

32. What is a target?

33. List the seven different targeting schemes used on commercially available ventilators.

A. _____

B. _____

C. _____

D. _____

E. _____

F. _____

G. _____

34. What are the three steps to classify a mode?

A. _____

B. _____

C. _____

TYPES OF VENTILATORS

35. Describe the volume and breath rate for conventional ventilation.

36. Describe some of the key features of the critical care ventilator.

37. Give four clinical reasons to use the noninvasive ventilator.

A. _____

B. _____

C. _____

D. _____

Copyright © 2025, Elsevier, Inc. All rights reserved.

A 21-year-old patient is placed on a ventilator following a closed head injury. The physician desires to control this patient's ventilation to achieve a specific CO_2 level in the arterial blood.

38. Would you select volume or pressure ventilation to best achieve this goal?

_____

39. Would you recommend a conventional ICU ventilator or a high-frequency option?

_____

WHAT DOES THE NBRC SAY?

Circle the best answer.

40. A resident asks you to identify which of the basic modes of ventilation on an ICU ventilator will permit spontaneous breathing for a patient with neuromuscular disease. You would select:
    1. CMV
    2. IMV
    3. CSV

    A. 1 and 3
    B. 1 and 2
    C. 2 and 3
    D. 1, 2, and 3

41. A patient in the early stages of ARDS is intubated. The physician states that he wishes to minimize the possibility of volutrauma or barotrauma. Which of the following modes would you recommend?
    A. Volume-controlled ventilation
    B. Manual ventilation
    C. CPAP
    D. Pressure-controlled ventilation

42. An 80-kg (176-lb) patient is being ventilated in a volume control mode. During a ventilator check, the therapist notes that the compliance has decreased from 40 ml/cm H_2O to 35 ml/cm H_2O. What effect will this change in compliance have on volume?
    A. No effect
    B. Increased minute volume
    C. Decreased minute volume
    D. Decreased tidal volume

FOOD FOR THOUGHT

What types of ventilators are your hospitals using? Does practice vary between community hospitals and trauma centers? Find out what ventilator your clinical site is using and become familiar with it prior to attending that site. A good starting point for the new therapist is to learn a lot about the modes that are most commonly used in current practice where you live and where you do your clinical training. The best RTs can make the best of whatever mode is used in their institution while acting as resources for the nurses and physicians. They pull the other modes out of their bag of tricks when the opportunity arises, *but only after making themselves experts*. Introducing a new ventilator or new mode of ventilation is fraught with hazards if in-service training doesn't come along with the change.

Copyright © 2025, Elsevier, Inc. All rights reserved.

47 Physiology of Ventilatory Support

WORD WIZARD

Look up the definitions in your glossary and write them out next to the words listed below.

1. Barotrauma _____

2. Time constant _____

3. Biotrauma _____

4. Transrespiratory pressure _____

5. Patient–ventilator asynchrony _____

6. Atelectrauma _____

7. Mean airway pressure _____

8. Transpulmonary pressure _____

PRESSURE AND PRESSURE GRADIENTS

9. Which pressure is responsible for maintaining normal alveolar inflation?

_____

10. Which pressure gradient is required to expand the lungs and chest wall together?

_____

11. Which pressure causes airflow in the airways?

_____

12. What happens to transpulmonary pressure during normal inspiration? Exhalation?

A. Inspiration _____

B. Exhalation _____

13. What happens to transpulmonary pressure during inspiration with a negative-pressure ventilator? During exhalation?

A. Inspiration _____

B. Exhalation _____

14. What is "tank shock?"

_____

15. What happens to the airway and pleural pressures during inspiration with a positive pressure ventilator?

_____

321

Copyright © 2025, Elsevier, Inc. All rights reserved.

Ventilation

16. A. What is the normal range of tidal volume during spontaneous breathing?
    B. What is the accepted tidal volume range for mechanical ventilation?

    A. _____ B. _____

17. Besides increasing the volume, how can you increase minute ventilation with the ventilator?

    _____

18. What effect does increasing the minute ventilation have on $PaCO_2$?

    _____

19. During spontaneous ventilation, where is gas mainly distributed? What about in positive pressure ventilation?

    A. Spontaneous _____

    B. PPV _____

20. How does perfusion, or blood flow, in the lung change during PPV?

    _____

Acid-Base Balance

21. Explain the importance of each the following as it relates to respiratory acidemia in a mechanically ventilated patient.

    A. Look at the patient _____

    B. Draw arterial blood _____

    C. Check electrolytes _____

    D. Check ECG _____

22. Explain the importance of each the following as it relates to respiratory alkalemia in a mechanically ventilated patient.

    A. Look at the patient _____

    B. Draw arterial blood _____

    C. Check electrolytes _____

    D. Check ECG _____

23. Explain the importance of each the following as it relates to metabolic acidemia and metabolic alkalemia in a mechanically ventilated patient.

    Metabolic acidemia

    A. Look at the patient _____

    B. Draw arterial blood _____

    Metabolic alkalemia

    A. Look at the patient _____

    B. Draw arterial blood _____

Copyright © 2025, Elsevier, Inc. All rights reserved.

Oxygenation

24. Explain how mechanical ventilation improves oxygenation for each of the following causes of hypoxemia:

A. Hypoventilation _____

B. $\dot{V}/\dot{Q}$ mismatch _____

C. Shunt _____

25. What range of F_IO_2 can a modern ICU ventilator deliver?

_____

26. State the formula for each of the following:

A. DO_2 _____

B. Alveolar air _____

C. Arterial oxygen content _____

D. Minute ventilation _____

LUNG MECHANICS

27. How long does it take for 95% of the alveoli in a normal lung to fill with air?

A. Time constants _____

B. Real time _____

What about 98% of alveoli? _____ 99%? _____

28. What are the two major factors that affect alveolar time constants?

A. _____

B. _____

29. You could help prolong the inspiratory phase for your patient with severe asthma by making the following adjustments:

A. Inspiratory time setting should be between _____seconds.

B. What is the primary limiting factor in the airway? _____

C. How could you resolve this limitation? _____

30. You could help prolong the expiratory phase for your COPD patient by making the following adjustments:

A. Inspiratory times should between _____seconds.

B. A common problem in these patients is _____because of long time constants.

C. Respiratory rates are typically _____.

31. What is meant by the term "peak inspiratory pressure?" What's the abbreviation?

_____

32. What is meant by the term "plateau pressure?" What's the symbol?

_____

323

Copyright © 2025, Elsevier, Inc. All rights reserved.

33. We can protect patient lungs from damage caused by pressure by maintaining plateau pressures at less than

_____ cm H$_2$O.

34. See if you know how to adjust mean airway pressure. Circle "T" for "true" if the choice is one that would *raise the mean airway pressure*. Circle "F" for false if it will not.
A. Increase peak pressure	T	F
B. Decrease inspiratory time	T	F
C. Synchronized IMV	T	F
D. Increase PEEP levels	T	F
E. Constant pressure pattern (PC mode, decelerating ramp flow)	T	F

35. How does increasing airway pressure affect the FRC and oxygenation?

A. FRC _____

B. Oxygenation _____

36. What will happen to compliance when too much PEEP is applied? Could you adjust the PEEP based on the changes

in compliance? _____

37. The pressure-volume curve is useful for establishing relationship of the lung-thorax in patients with ARDS. Name each of the following:

A. Lower inflection point: _____ or _____

B. Upper inflection point: _____

38. Why does dead space increase during mechanical ventilation?

_____

Work of Breathing

39. Work of breathing (WOB) consists of what two components?

A. _____

B. _____

40. Measuring WOB at the bedside is difficult. What is normal WOB? What three variables does the experienced therapist use to determine whether WOB is excessive?

Normal WOB: _____

A. _____

B. _____

C. _____

PULMONARY EFFECTS OF POSITIVE PRESSURE MECHANICAL VENTILATION

41. List two negative pulmonary effects of too much PEEP.

A. _____

B. _____

Copyright © 2025, Elsevier, Inc. All rights reserved.

42. Why can PEEP be a problem with severe unilateral lung disease?

43. Compare square flow patterns with descending ramp.

PHYSIOLOGIC EFFECTS OF VENTILATORY MODES

44. Identify two potential harmful effects of inappropriate trigger-level setting when a patient's ventilation is in CMV mode.

    A. _____

    B. _____

45. When is VC-CMV indicated?

    _____

46. When would you choose PC-CMV over VC-CMV?

    _____

47. What are the possible benefits of APRV?

    _____

48. When is PSV useful?

    _____

49. Bilevel PAP was originally developed for treatment of obstructive sleep apnea. It has also been shown to be useful in acute care setting with COPD exacerbations. Explain.

    _____

50. How does proportional-assist ventilation (PAV) work?

    _____

51. Compare PAV to neutrally adjusted ventilatory assist (NAVA).

    _____

    _____

    _____

Copyright © 2025, Elsevier, Inc. All rights reserved.

52. Automatic tube compensation is not a mode of ventilation. What is it really? What does the RT input?

_____

_____

_____

53. How is patient-ventilator interaction monitored in adaptive control/dual control mode?

Patient Positioning to Optimize Oxygenation and Ventilation

54. What group of patients is most likely to benefit from prone positioning?

55. What should be monitored when changing positioning of patients?

_____

CARDIOVASCULAR EFFECTS OF POSITIVE PRESSURE MECHANICAL VENTILATION

56. Briefly explain the negative effects of PPV on the heart. What is this effect dependent on?

_____

57. How can you use the ventilator to temporarily manage increased ICP?

_____

58. Explain the mechanism behind the drop in urine output in ventilated patients.

A. Direct _____

B. Indirect _____

59. Why is sedation necessary for the management of a patient in the ICU?

Copyright © 2025, Elsevier, Inc. All rights reserved.

60. When using a chest cuirass and poncho-type negative-pressure ventilators, what problems can result in hypoventilation?

    A. _____

    B. _____

61. Positive pressure ventilation has long been associated with barotrauma. List three of the clinical signs of pneumothorax.

    A. Chest motion _____

    B. Percussion note _____

    C. Breath sounds _____

62. Tension pneumothorax is life threatening in a ventilated patient. How and where is this treated?

    A. How?

    B. Where in the chest?

63. What is volutrauma, and how is it prevented?

64. Oxygen toxicity may damage lung tissue. Every effort should be made to reduce the F_IO_2 to what value?

    _____

65. List three ways to reduce the risk of ventilator-associated pneumonias.

    A. Positioning _____

    B. Endotracheal tubes _____

    C. Reduce condensates _____

Copyright © 2025, Elsevier, Inc. All rights reserved.

66. What are two positive physiologic effects of PPV?

67. Research indicates what type of flow pattern is better for ventilator synchrony and gas exchange?

68. What type of triggering appears to be a better choice when it is available on the ventilator?

69. Why is PEEP applied in restrictive disease? Why is PEEP applied in obstructive disease?

CASE STUDY

Case 1, Part 1

A trauma patient is stabilized after a motor vehicle accident. He is intubated and transported to the ICU, where you place him on a ventilator. As soon as you put him on the machine, his blood pressure falls dramatically.

70. What should you do (right away!)?

_____

71. What is the most likely cause of hypotension in a trauma patient who has been placed on positive pressure ventilation?

_____

Copyright © 2025, Elsevier, Inc. All rights reserved.

Two days later, the patient has developed poor lung compliance and hypoxemia associated with noncardiogenic pulmonary edema (ARDS). He is being ventilated on VC-CMV, frequency of 12, tidal volume of 700 mL, +15 cm H_2O PEEP, and F_IO_2 0.70. Blood gases show pH 7.37, $PaCO_2$ 38, and PaO_2 55. Peak inspiratory pressure is 60 cm H_2O, and plateau pressure is 50 cm H_2O.

72. There are two serious problems here. Identify them.

    A. Serious problem No. 1 _____

    B. Serious problem No. 2 _____

73. What change(s) in ventilator strategy would you suggest?
    A. Problem No. 1

    B. Problem No. 2

WHAT DOES THE NBRC SAY?

Review each of the common modes of ventilation. You will be asked questions to make sure you really know your modes.

FOOD FOR THOUGHT

74. If the newest modes of ventilation are not proven to alter patient outcomes, why should we use them?

75. Patients on ventilators have a high incidence of GI bleeding. Why is GI bleeding such a big deal to RTs?

329

Copyright © 2025, Elsevier, Inc. All rights reserved.

48 Patient-Ventilator Interactions

WORD WIZARD

State the cause for each of the following terms and how you would correct the problem.

1. Missed triggering

   A. Cause: _____

   B. Modification to correct: _____

2. Double triggering

   A. Cause: _____

   B. Modification to correct: _____

3. Auto-triggering

   A. Cause: _____

   B. Modification to correct: _____

4. Reverse triggering

   A. Cause: _____

   B. Modification to correct: _____

5. Delayed triggering

   A. Cause: _____

   B. Modification to correct: _____

6. Mode asynchrony

   A. Cause: _____

   B. Modification to correct: _____

7. Cycle asynchrony

   A. Cause: _____

   B. Modification to correct: _____

EFFECT OF POOR PATIENT-VENTILATOR INTERACTION ON OUTCOME

8. What is patient-ventilator interaction and why is it critical during mechanical ventilation?

Copyright © 2025, Elsevier, Inc. All rights reserved.

9. How can poor patient-ventilator interactions negatively affect the patient?

10. List four issues with an artificial airway that can cause poor patient-ventilator interaction.

    A. _____

    B. _____

    C. _____

    D. _____

11. List three problems that can cause rapid deterioration in the patients' clinical status.

    A. _____

    B. _____

    C. _____

VARIABLES CONTROLLED DURING MECHANICAL VENTILATION

12. Why are the modes proportional assist ventilation (PAV) and neutrally adjusted ventilatory assist (NAVA) least likely to cause asynchrony?

13. In PAV and NAVA, what happens when patient effort increases?

TYPES OF ASYNCHRONY

14. When does flow asynchrony occur? Is there a mode in which it is more likely to occur?

15. What must you do to prevent flow asynchrony?

16. In which two modes of ventilation is mode asynchrony least likely to occur?

    A. _____

    B. _____

17. In which mode of mechanical ventilation is cycle asynchrony most likely to occur? Why?

331

Copyright © 2025, Elsevier, Inc. All rights reserved.

18. What is a targeting scheme?

19. Describe the targeting schemes listed below.
    A. Set-point (s):

    B. Dual (d):

    C. Bio-variable (b):

    D. Servo (r):

    E. Adaptive (a):

    F. Optimal (o):

    G. Intelligent (i):

Copyright © 2025, Elsevier, Inc. All rights reserved.

20. What does the term *Mode TAG* refer to?

21. How are patient-ventilator interactions (PVI) evaluated?

WHAT DOES THE NBRC SAY?

22. A respiratory therapist determined a patient receiving mechanical ventilation developed auto-PEEP due to dynamic airflow obstruction. Which of the following should the therapist do?
    A. Add an inspiratory plateau.
    B. Add mechanical dead space.
    C. Decrease the mandatory rate.
    D. Decrease the inspiratory flow.

23. The following data are obtained for a patient who is receiving VC ventilation with a VT of 400 mL:

	0600	0900
Peak airway pressure	32 cm H_2O	45 cm H_2O
Plateau pressure	25 cm H_2O	25 cm H_2O

This information indicates
    A. increased air trapping.
    B. increased airways resistance.
    C. decreased inspiratory flow.
    D. decreased static compliance.

24. A basketball tournament is in town, and a 6 foot 11 inch male player was injured in a motor vehicle crash following a championship party. His is intubated and receiving mechanical ventilation when you assess him and notice he is double triggering the ventilator. What is the most likely cause?
    A. The patient's is desiring a larger breath than is set on the ventilator.
    B. The flow from the ventilator does not match the flow demand of the patient.
    C. The length of time between the beginning of the patient's inspiration and activation of the ventilator is excessive.
    D. The ventilator ends the breath at a time different from when the patient's respiratory center wants to end the breath.

FOOD FOR THOUGHT

Mechanical ventilation is not a cookie-cutter modality. There is no one mode or one setting that will ensure the most appropriate patient-ventilator interaction occurs. The only thing that makes a difference is how the RT manages the patient!

Copyright © 2025, Elsevier, Inc. All rights reserved.

49 Initiating and Adjusting Invasive Ventilatory Support

CASE STUDIES

Let's go right to the cases and find out if you understand how to initiate and adjust ventilatory support. This chapter will use case studies to help you understand how to initiate and adjust invasive ventilatory support. Five basic types of lungs and 10 specific disorders can account for almost every case of mechanical ventilation.

Case 1

A 5-foot 5-inch, 60-kg (132-lb) young woman attempted suicide by drug overdose. She is unconscious and breathing slowly and shallowly. The emergency physician elects to intubate this patient.

1. What size ET tube would be appropriate for an adult female?
    A. 6.0-mm inside diameter
    B. 7.0-mm outside diameter
    C. 7.5-mm inside diameter
    D. 8.0-mm inside diameter

2. In the emergency setting, how will you assess proper tube placement?
    1. Auscultate the chest.
    2. Auscultate the epigastrium.
    3. Attach an exhaled O_2 monitor.
    4. Observe chest wall motion.

    A. 1 and 2
    B. 1 and 3
    C. 2, 3, and 4
    D. 1, 2, and 4

After the intubation is completed, a small amount of white secretions are suctioned from the airway. The physician requests a room air ABG at this point. Results show:

pH	7.25
$PaCO_2$	60 mm Hg
PaO_2	55 mm Hg
HCO_3^-	26 mEq/L

Vital signs are:

HR	115
BP	125/75
RR	26
Temp	37

Copyright © 2025, Elsevier, Inc. All rights reserved.

A chest film is taken, which reveals the tip of the endotracheal tube to be 4 cm above the carina with no sign of a pneumothorax.

3. What action would you recommend in regard to the ET tube placement?
   A. Advance the tube 2 to 3 cm.
   B. Withdraw the tube 2 to 3 cm.
   C. Maintain current placement.
   D. Remove the tube and insert a laryngeal mask airway.

4. The ABG results are interpreted as _____.
   A. metabolic acidosis with severe hypoxemia
   B. respiratory acidosis with moderate hypoxemia
   C. partially compensated respiratory alkalosis with mild hypoxemia
   D. partially compensated metabolic alkalosis with moderate hypoxemia

The patient is transported to the ICU. The physician requests that you initiate mechanical ventilation.

5. Calculate predicted body weight.
   A. 45 kg
   B. 59 kg
   C. 65 kg
   D. 130 kg

6. Which of the following volumes would you recommend?
   A. 410 ml
   B. 610 ml
   C. 710 ml
   D. 810 ml

7. What mode and rate would you select?
   A. PSV, 10 cmH$_2$O
   B. VC-IMV, 6
   C. VC-CMV, 12
   D. VC-CMV, 22

8. What type of humidification system would you recommend for this patient?
   A. Heated wick humidifier set at 35°C
   B. HME
   C. Heated passover humidifier
   D. Bubble humidifier

Three days later, the patient is alert, and weaning is initiated. When the rate is decreased to 5, however, the patient's spontaneous respiratory rate rises to 30 and tidal volumes drop to 200 ml.

9. To help resolve this problem you might recommend initiation of _____.
   A. CMV
   B. AC
   C. PSV
   D. APRV

Copyright © 2025, Elsevier, Inc. All rights reserved.

Paramedics bring a 5-foot 2-inch, 50-kg (110-lb) 65-year-old woman with a history of COPD to the emergency department for treatment of dyspnea. She is wearing a nasal cannula set at 2 L/min. ABGs are drawn. Results show

pH	7.30
$PaCO_2$	70 mm Hg
PaO_2	45 mm Hg
HCO_3^-	34 mEq/L

Vital signs are

HR	100
BP	100/70
RR	34
Temp	39

Noninvasive positive pressure breathing is attempted with bilevel ventilation, but the patient is unable to tolerate the mask and fights the system. A decision is made to intubate and initiate mechanical ventilation. The patient is given a small amount of sedation and intubated nasally with a 6.5-mm ID tube. Settings are

Mode	VC-IMV
Rate	14
V_T	400 ml
F_IO_2	0.28
PEEP	0
Peak flow	20 LPM
Flow pattern	Decelerating ramp
Sensitivity	1.5 cm H_2O below baseline

10. How long should you wait before drawing an ABG to assess the results of these settings?
    A. 5 minutes
    B. 20 minutes
    C. 40 minutes
    D. 60 minutes

11. What is the maximum desirable plateau pressure during mechanical ventilation?
    A. 15 cm H_2O
    B. 25 cm H_2O
    C. 28 cm H_2O
    D. 40 cm H_2O

During your first patient-ventilator system assessment the following observations are made.

PIP	40 cm H_2O
Plateau	35 cm H_2O
Set rate	14
Total rate	25
Exhaled V_T	425 ml
I:E ratio	1:1.5

12. What high-pressure alarm limit should you set?
    A. 35 cm H_2O
    B. 45 cm H_2O
    C. 50 cm H_2O
    D. 65 cm H_2O

Copyright © 2025, Elsevier, Inc. All rights reserved.

13. What value should you set for the low-minute ventilation alarm?
    A. 2.0 L
    B. 3.0 L
    C. 4.0 L
    D. 5.0 L

14. Which of the following would result in a lower work of breathing for this patient?
    1. Addition of 100 ml mechanical dead space
    2. Initiation of PSV at 5 cm H_2O
    3. Changing to flow-triggering 2 L/min
    4. Addition of 10 cm H_2O PEEP

    A. 1 and 2 only
    B. 2 and 3 only
    C. 1 and 3 only
    D. 2, 3, and 4

15. What action should you take to increase the I:E ratio?
    A. Increase the peak flow.
    B. Increase the tidal volume.
    C. Increase the set rate.
    D. Increase the F_IO_2.

16. What I:E ratio would provide sufficient time for exhalation and prevent auto-PEEP in this COPD patient?
    A. 1:1
    B. 1:2
    C. 1:4
    D. 1:10

Case 3

A 5-foot 6-inch woman who weighs 100 kg (220 lb) is in the ICU following surgery for multiple injuries sustained in a motor vehicle accident. She has an arterial line and a pulmonary artery catheter in place. Her chest radiograph shows bilateral infiltrates consistent with ARDS. The ET tube is in good position.

Current ventilator settings are:

Mode	VC- CMV
V_T	800
Rate	12
F_IO_2	0.70
PEEP	5 cm H_2O
Peak flow	60 L/min, decelerating ramp
Sensitivity	1.0 cm H_2O below baseline

17. What is this patient's approximate predicted body weight?
    A. 50 kg
    B. 60 kg
    C. 80 kg
    D. 100 kg

18. What initial tidal volume would you recommend to prevent further lung injury?
    A. 460 ml
    B. 660 ml
    C. 720 ml
    D. Maintain current setting

Copyright © 2025, Elsevier, Inc. All rights reserved.

The following data are obtained:

HR	110, NSR with occasional PVCs
BP	110/75 mm Hg
SpO_2	88%
PA	38/8 mm Hg
PCWP	12 mm Hg
CO	5.8 L/min
SvO_2	59%

19. With regard to the patient's oxygenation, what action would you recommend?
    A. Increase the F_IO_2.
    B. Increase the PEEP.
    C. Add mechanical dead space.
    D. Maintain current settings.

A PEEP trial is conducted with the following results.

PEEP	Cstat	PaO_2	CO
5	22	57	5.8
10	25	66	5.7
15	30	72	5.9
20	25	77	5.2
25	22	85	4.8

20. What PEEP level would you recommend?
    A. 5
    B. 10
    C. 15
    D. 20
    E. 25

The patient continues to deteriorate over the next 2 days. Her compliance and PaO_2 have decreased, while PIP has increased to 60 cm H_2O to maintain a normal $PaCO_2$.

21. Which of the following ventilator modes could be considered as alternatives?
    1. PC-CMV
    2. VC-IMV
    3. APRV
    4. CPAP

    A. 1 and 3 only
    B. 2 and 3 only
    C. 2 and 4 only
    D. 1 and 4 only

22. Which of these techniques are used with ARDS with a P/F ratio less than 100 to reduce lung injury or improve oxygenation?
    1. Expiratory retard
    2. Prone positioning
    3. Permissive hypercapnia
    4. Unilateral lung ventilation

    A. 1 and 2
    B. 2 and 3
    C. 1 and 4
    D. 3 and 4

Copyright © 2025, Elsevier, Inc. All rights reserved.

A respiratory student who fell down the stairs while reading *Egan's* suffered a closed-head injury. The student is 5 feet 5 inches tall and weighs 60 kg. ICP and blood pressure are elevated. She is being ventilated with these settings.

Mode   VC-CMV
Rate   10
V_T 600
F_IO_2 .30
PEEP   0

Blood gases on these settings are:

pH   7.40
$PaCO_2$ 40
PaO_2 55
HCO_3^- 24

23. This blood gas should be interpreted as _____.
   A. normal with moderate hypoxemia
   B. respiratory alkalosis with mild hypoxemia
   C. compensated respiratory acidosis with severe hypoxemia
   D. compensated metabolic alkalosis with moderate hypoxemia

24. With regard to the oxygenation, what change would you suggest?
   A. Increase the PEEP.
   B. Increase the rate.
   C. Change to APRV.
   D. Increase the F_IO_2.

25. With regard to the ventilation, what change would you suggest?
   A. Increase the rate.
   B. Increase the tidal volume.
   C. Change to IMV.
   D. Add mechanical dead space.

26. What is the formula for calculating the rate needed to produce a desired change in $PaCO_2$?
   A. $PaCO_2$ measured × set rate ÷ $PaCO_2$ desired
   B. $PaCO_2$ desired × set rate ÷ $PaCO_2$ measured
   C. $PaCO_2$ measured × $PaCO_2$ desired ÷ set rate
   D. $PaCO_2$ measured × PaO_2 measured ÷ set rate

27. What rate would you suggest for this patient if the desired $PaCO_2$ is 30 mm Hg?
   A. 8
   B. 10
   C. 14
   D. 18

28. How long should you maintain a head injury patient in a hyperventilated state?
   A. 2 to 4 hours
   B. 6 to 8 hours
   C. 12 to 24 hours
   D. 24 to 48 hours

Copyright © 2025, Elsevier, Inc. All rights reserved.

A 5-foot 7-inch, 27-year-old woman who weighs 140 lb with a long history of asthma including previous intubation and mechanical ventilation presents in the emergency department with high-pitched, diffuse wheezing. She is barely able to talk because of her dyspnea. She has not responded to two consecutive SVN treatments with 5 mg of albuterol and 0.5 mg of Atrovent. Peak flows are not measurable, and SpO_2 is 92% on 2 L via nasal cannula. She is using her accessory muscles to breathe and has some intercostal retractions on inspiration. She is started on IV Solu-Medrol, continuous bronchodilator therapy, and ECG monitoring. One hour later, she is lethargic, and breath sounds are virtually absent. You draw an ABG with the following results:

pH	7.29
$PaCO_2$	55 mm Hg
PaO_2	64 mm Hg
HCO_3^-	24 mmol
SaO_2	90%

29. What action would you recommend at this time?
    A. Continuation of present therapy
    B. Oral intubation with 7.5 ET tube and mechanical ventilation
    C. Trial of NIV via bilevel mask ventilation
    D. Tracheostomy and mechanical ventilation

30. The emergency physician elects to move the patient to the MICU as soon as she is stabilized. You assist in the transport. In the ICU, you are asked to set up the ventilator. You would select:
    A. VC-IMV 14, 400, 0.40 F_IO_2, +3 PEEP, +5 PSV
    B. VC-CMV 12, 350, +5 PEEP, 0.40 F_IO_2
    C. APRV high PEEP 30, low PEEP 0, 0.60 F_IO_2, 1-second release time
    D. PSV 10 cmH_2O, 0.30 F_IO_2

31. What pharmacologic agent is recommended at this time?
    A. Inhaled corticosteroids
    B. Sedation with midazolam
    C. Paralysis with cisatracurium besylate
    D. Respiratory stimulus with doxapram

32. Which of the following are major concerns when ventilating severe asthmatics?
    1. Pulmonary barotrauma
    2. Development of auto-PEEP
    3. Ventilator asynchrony
    4. High airway pressures

    A. 1 and 2
    B. 1, 3, and 4
    C. 2, 3, and 4
    D. 1, 2, 3, and 4

33. An appropriate peak flow and flow pattern for this patient would include
    A. 40 L/min with a decelerating flow waveform.
    B. 20 L/min with a square flow waveform.
    C. 100 L/min with a sine wave flow pattern.
    D. 50 L/min with an accelerating flow waveform.

34. What alteration to the mode of ventilation might be useful to prevent barotrauma and improve comfort?
    A. Addition of mechanical dead space
    B. Using a heated humidifier
    C. Switching to pressure control
    D. Utilizing inverse ratio ventilation

Copyright © 2025, Elsevier, Inc. All rights reserved.

Case 6

A 6-foot, 176-lb 66-year-old man has been brought to the SICU following coronary artery bypass graft surgery. He has no history of lung disease. He is intubated with a No. 8 oral ET tube. The anesthesiologist asks you to select ventilator settings.

35. What tidal volume is appropriate for this postoperative patient?
    A. 550 ml
    B. 660 ml
    C. 800 ml
    D. 950 ml

36. Why should you add PEEP to the system?
    A. To prevent auto-PEEP
    B. To prevent atelectasis
    C. To prevent cardiogenic pulmonary edema
    D. To prevent barotrauma

37. What is your primary goal for this patient?
    A. Prevent ventilator-associated barotrauma.
    B. Prevent ventilator-associated pneumonia.
    C. Control air trapping.
    D. Wean and extubate as quickly as possible.

WHAT DOES THE NBRC SAY?

Circle the best answer.

38. A patient with CHF is placed on the ventilator with proper tube placement confirmed. The respiratory therapist should
    A. obtain a sputum sample for culture.
    B. assess changes in intracranial pressure.
    C. assess changes in blood pressure.
    D. obtain a chest x-ray.

39. A patient is receiving mechanical ventilation via VC- CMV with a mandatory rate of 14. Peak inspiratory pressures are in the low 50s. The physician wants to maintain the mean airway pressure but lower the peak pressure. What would you recommend?
    A. Increase the mandatory rate.
    B. Increase the inspiratory flow.
    C. Initiate pressure-controlled ventilation.
    D. Initiate IMV with pressure support.

40. What is an appropriate range for respiratory rate (f) when using high-frequency oscillation ventilation in adults?
    A. 1-2 Hz
    B. 3-5 Hz
    C. 10-15 Hz
    D. 20-30 Hz

41. A patient with ARDS due to trauma from a motor vehicle crash is placed on mechanical ventilation. The man is 182 cm (6 feet) tall and weights 100 kg (220 lb). With respect to ventilator settings, what tidal volume would you recommend?
    A. 460 ml
    B. 560 ml
    C. 660 ml
    D. 800 ml

Copyright © 2025, Elsevier, Inc. All rights reserved.

42. An apneic patient is placed on mechanical ventilation following surgery. What range of rates is typical for initiating mechanical ventilation on an adult patient?
    A. 4-8
    B. 8-12
    C. 12-16
    D. 16-20

43. A patient is being mechanically ventilated in CMV mode. When the patient begins to inhale, airway pressure drops to –4 cm H_2O below baseline before a breath is started. What control needs to be adjusted?
    A. Frequency
    B. PEEP
    C. Pressure support
    D. Sensitivity

44. A patient with ARDS is being mechanically ventilated with a PEEP of 10 cm H_2O and an F_IO_2 of 0.80. When the patient is removed from the ventilator for suctioning, he experiences decreased oxygen saturation and increased heart rate. What should the respiratory therapist recommend?
    A. Decreasing the PEEP to 5 cm H_2O
    B. Changing to a closed suction system
    C. Giving SVN with albuterol 2.5 mg
    D. Increasing the F_IO_2 on the ventilator

45. A 70-kg patient is ventilated on VC-IMV mode with a rate of 8, tidal volume of 700, F_IO_2 of 0.40, PEEP of 4 cm H_2O, pressure support of 4 cm H_2O, and an inspiratory flow rate of 45 L/min. The patient is breathing 22 times per minute in between the machine breaths with a tidal volume of 150 ml. What change should the respiratory therapist recommend?
    A. Increasing the peak inspiratory flow rate
    B. Increasing the respiratory rate
    C. Increasing the set tidal volume
    D. Increasing the pressure support

46. A 50-kg adult female is mechanically ventilated following a cardiac arrest. What tidal volume setting is recommended for this patient?
    A. 250 ml
    B. 350 ml
    C. 450 ml
    D. 550 ml

47. Initiation of an expiratory hold facilitates the measurement of
    A. plateau pressure.
    B. auto-PEEP.
    C. peak airway pressure.
    D. set PEEP.

48. You are ventilating a patient in a pressure-controlled mode of ventilation. The patient is not obtaining the desired minute ventilation. What would you suggest to fix this issue?
    A. Increase the inspiratory pressure limit.
    B. Increase the tidal volume.
    C. Increase the set frequency.
    D. Increase the flow rate.

Copyright © 2025, Elsevier, Inc. All rights reserved.

49. What driving pressures have recently been linked to increase in mortality rates in patients with ARDS?

50. What are the common ventilator modes where you are training or working? Practice them in the lab.

Copyright © 2025, Elsevier, Inc. All rights reserved.

50 Noninvasive Ventilation

INDICATIONS FOR NONINVASIVE VENTILATION

1. What is the primary goal of noninvasive ventilation (NIV)?

2. List three potential benefits of NIV in the acute care setting.

    A. _____

    B. _____

    C. _____

3. In the acute care setting, NIV is indicated for numerous conditions. List at least four.

    A. _____

    B. _____

    C. _____

    D. _____

4. NIV is also indicated for the long-term care setting. List four conditions.

    A. _____

    B. _____

    C. _____

    D. _____

SELECTING APPROPRIATE PATIENTS FOR NONINVASIVE VENTILATION

5. How is the need for ventilatory assistance established?

    A. Respiratory rate _____

    B. Dyspnea _____

    C. $PaCO_2$ and pH _____

    D. P/F ratio _____

Copyright © 2025, Elsevier, Inc. All rights reserved.

6. List at least four exclusion criteria for NIV.

   A. _____

   B. _____

   C. _____

   D. _____

7. What is the standard of care for acute COPD exacerbation or cardiogenic pulmonary edema in the acute care setting?

   _____

8. Compare CPAP to bilevel noninvasive ventilation in the treatment of acute cardiogenic pulmonary edema. When does bilevel outperform CPAP?

   _____

9. Describe the two basic parts of the decision-making process for a patient with chronic restrictive thoracic disease.

   A.

   B.

EQUIPMENT USED FOR NONINVASIVE VENTILATION

10. What is an interface?

    _____

11. Which type of patient interface is most commonly used for NIV? Which is usually the best choice for treating patients in acute respiratory failure?

    _____

12. What is the key factor in patient tolerance and NIV efficacy?

    _____

13. Compare nasal mask sizing and oronasal mask sizing techniques. Which is more susceptible to leaks?

    _____

Copyright © 2025, Elsevier, Inc. All rights reserved.

14. List three disadvantages associated with oronasal masks.

    A. _____

    B. _____

    C. _____

15. Patients with what complication would benefit from a total face mask?

    _____

Types of Mechanical Ventilators and Modes of Ventilation

16. Define the following terms:

    A. CPAP:

    B. IPAP:

    C. EPAP:

17. What happens to tidal volume when you increase the EPAP without increasing the IPAP?

    _____

18. What are some of the problems with using critical care ventilators to deliver mask ventilation? What may help?

19. How can you recognize active exhalation on the ventilator's graphics?

20. What are two ways to correct the problem of active exhalation?

    A. _____

    B. _____

21. List two advantageous performance characteristics of home care ventilators.

    A. _____

    B. _____

22. What is the temperature for heated humidity when using NIV? Why is it used?

Copyright © 2025, Elsevier, Inc. All rights reserved.

23. How should your patient be positioned when applying NIV?

24. How should you prepare the patient for the experience?

25. What pressure could open the esophagus?

26. What tidal volumes are you aiming for when applying NIV? Which control do you adjust if the volume is too low?

    A. Goal: _____

    B. Adjust: _____

27. Which two adjustments can be made to improve oxygenation?

28. Fill in the chart below regarding possible side effects and complications of NIV.

	Possible Solutions
Interface-Related Side Effects	
Discomfort	
Erythema	
Claustrophobia	
Pressure ulcer	
Skin rash	
Air–Pressure-Related or Flow-Related Side Effects	
Nasal congestion	
Nasal dryness	
Sinus or ear pain	
Eye irritation	
Gastric distention	
Serious Complications	
Aspiration	
Pneumothorax	
Hypotension	

347

Copyright © 2025, Elsevier, Inc. All rights reserved.

Mary Mac is a 61-year-old female with a 60-pack-year history of smoking who was diagnosed with COPD 7 years ago. She is currently being treated on the general floor for community-acquired pneumonia. She has been intubated twice because of exacerbation of COPD and is currently complaining of dyspnea. Vital signs are heart rate 96 beats/min, blood pressure 138/86 mm Hg, respiratory rate 22 breaths/min, and SpO_2 90% on a nasal cannula at 6 L/min. ABGs reveal pH 7.25, $PaCO_2$ 66 mmHg, PaO_2 59 mmHg. She is very anxious and tripoding.

29. What treatment would you initiate at this time?

30. What is your goal with your care of Mary Mac?

31. Where would you initiate the treatment you choose?

Mary is now stable and is requiring Atrovent.

32. Can this be given if she is currently receiving NIV? If yes, where would you position the nebulizer? Where would you position an MDI?

33. She has been on NIV 3 hours and Mary Mac is not improving. What treatment would you suggest to the physician?

WHAT DOES THE NBRC SAY?

Questions 34-37 refer to the following scenario. Circle the best answer.

A 60-kg, 70-year-old patient with COPD does not wish to be intubated and has an advance directive supporting his wishes. The patient is admitted to the medical ICU in respiratory failure. ABGs reveal pH 7.25, $PaCO_2$ 66 mm Hg, and PaO_2 50 mm Hg.

34. What mode of therapy would the respiratory therapist recommend in this situation?
    A. Nasal cannula at 6 L/min
    B. Nonrebreathing mask at 10 L/min
    C. Continuous positive airway pressure (CPAP)
    D. Noninvasive ventilation (NIV)

35. NIV is initiated on spontaneous mode with F_1O_2 0.40, IPAP of 8 cm H_2O, and EPAP of 2 cm H_2O. ABGs reveal pH 7.29, $PaCO_2$ 54, PaO_2 52, and HCO_3 30. The respiratory therapist should recommend what change in regard to the carbon dioxide levels?
    A. Increase the respiratory rate setting.
    B. Increase the tidal volume setting.
    C. Increase the IPAP.
    D. Increase the EPAP.

Copyright © 2025, Elsevier, Inc. All rights reserved.

36. What should the RT recommend to improve oxygenation?
    A. Increase the respiratory rate setting.
    B. Increase the tidal volume setting.
    C. Increase the IPAP.
    D. Increase the EPAP.

37. What exhaled tidal volume would you target for this patient?
    A. 200 ml
    B. 350 ml
    C. 475 ml
    D. 600 ml

38. A patient is brought into the ED with hypoxemia associated with severe cardiogenic hypoxemia. The patient has a respiratory rate of 24, heart rate of 126, and a blood pressure of 68/40. What mode of therapy would the respiratory therapist recommend in this situation?
    A. Noninvasive ventilation (NIV) with BiPAP
    B. Nonrebreathing mask at 15 L/min
    C. Continuous positive airway pressure (CPAP)
    D. Intubation and invasive ventilation

39. A 29-year-old patient who is morbidly obese is admitted to the ED with a productive cough, fever, and shortness of breath. The patient's vital signs are stable and he is awake and alert. After initiation of bronchodilator therapy and antibiotics, results for serial blood gas analyses reveal:

	7:00 AM	8:00 AM
F_1O	0.21	0.50
pH	7.28	7.22
$PaCO_2$	72 mmHg	85 mmHg
PaO_2	45 mmHg	56 mmHg
HCO_3^-	34 mEq/L	35 mEq/L
BE	+5 mEq/L	+4 mEq/L
SaO_2	80%	89%

The patient's clinical condition remains unchanged and the physician asks for suggestions in therapy. Which of the following should a respiratory therapist recommend?
    A. Intubation and invasive ventilation.
    B. Initiate non-invasive ventilation.
    C. Decrease F_1O_2 to 0.45.
    D. Maintain current therapy.

FOOD FOR THOUGHT

40. As an RT you should always be your patient's advocate. The last thing you should want to do is intubate and mechanically ventilate a patient. If you have to, you should always be thinking of how to get patients off the ventilator and breathing on their own again. Your knowledge and understanding of NIV and cardiopulmonary pathophysiology can help. So, study, read, and learn! Your patients are depending on it.

Copyright © 2025, Elsevier, Inc. All rights reserved.

51 Extracorporeal Life Support

Word Wizard

Match the following terms with their definitions as they relate to extracorporeal life support.

_____ Venous reservoir

_____ Sweep flow

_____ VA ECMO

_____ Pump flow

_____ VV ECMO

_____ Hybrid ECMO

_____ Activated clotting time

_____ ECCO2R

A. The primary test for anticoagulation at the bedside.
B. ECMO that involves extra drainage or return cannulas.
C. Support is partial cardiopulmonary bypass, providing both cardiac and pulmonary support.
D. The bladder.
E. Dependent on the patient's preload and afterload.
F. Gas flow.
G. Only provides pulmonary support.
H. The removal of carbon dioxide as opposed to the delivery of oxygen

EXTRACORPOREAL LIFE SUPPORT (ECLS)

1. What are the primary goals of extracorporeal membrane oxygenation (ECMO)?

2. What are the four types of ECMO?

   A. _____

   B. _____

   C. _____

   D. _____

3. Describe the qualities that make an RT a prime candidate as an ECMO specialist.

4. What two ways is ECMO primarily used in the pediatric and adult patient?

   A. _____

   B. _____

5. Describe normal cardiopulmonary physiology during circulation of the blood beginning in the right heart.

Copyright © 2025, Elsevier, Inc. All rights reserved.

6. What two components make up the total oxygen content in the blood?

    A. _____

    B. _____

ECMO EQUIPMENT

7. ECMO equipment has what task?

8. Describe an ECMO circuit. Is short or long tubing best?

9. Why is tubing length particularly important in the newborn population?

10. When blood is drained from the patient, where does it go?

11. How is the ECMO system powered?

12. What three situations can cause excessive negative pressure on the right atrium?

    A. _____

    B. _____

    C. _____

13. When adjusting the blender, what are the saturation and PO_2 goals for the hemoglobin leaving the oxygenator?

14. Why does CO_2 diffuse into the sweep fibers?

15. How does sweep flow relate to CO_2 elimination?

16. What is a typical sweep flow to pump flow ratio?

17. What additional ECMO equipment is needed?

ANTICOAGULATION MANAGEMENT ON ECMO

18. What is the most common medication used as an anticoagulant during ECMO?

Copyright © 2025, Elsevier, Inc. All rights reserved.

19. List three factors that can affect the activated clotting time (ACT) in ECMO patients.

A. _____

B. _____

C. _____

20. What does the "M" number mean as it relates to cannulas?

21. What three characteristics are considered when sizing cannulas?

A. _____

B. _____

C. _____

TYPES OF SUPPORT

22. Give a detailed explanation for each of the following types of ECMO.

A. VV ECMO _____

B. VA ECMO _____

C. ECCO2R _____

D. Hybrid ECMO _____

23. How many cannulas need to be placed for VA ECMO? Where are they placed?

24. Give indications for each of the following types of ECMO.

A. VV ECMO _____

B. VA ECMO _____

C. ECCO2R _____

D. Hybrid ECMO _____

25. Give a disadvantage VA ECMO.

26. What advantages does VV ECMO have over VA ECMO?

A. _____

27. List six physiologic complications of ECMO.

A. _____

B. _____

C. _____

D. _____

E. _____

F. _____

Copyright © 2025, Elsevier, Inc. All rights reserved.

WEANING AND DECANNULATION FROM ECMO

28. Describe the weaning process for VA and VV ECMO. Include mechanical ventilator parameters.

    A. VA _____

    B. VV _____

SUMMARY CHECKLIST

29. What is a major advantage of ECMO as it relates to ventilatory support?

30. Why is anticoagulant therapy necessary during ECMO?

FOOD FOR THOUGHT

An RT's role in patient care is becoming more and more advanced, so read the literature and get ready!

Copyright © 2025, Elsevier, Inc. All rights reserved.

52 Monitoring the Patient in the Intensive Care Unit

The best monitor is a knowledgeable, observant, and dedicated health care professional.
Donald F. Egan, MD

WORD WIZARD

Match these key terms to the definitions that follow.

Terms	Definitions
1. _____ Afterload	A. Pressure the ventricle has to contract against.
	B. Pressure stretching the ventricle at the onset of contraction.
2. _____ Swan-Ganz catheter	C. Unreal events seen on monitors often caused by movement.
	D. Popular system for measuring neurologic impairment.
3. _____ Q_s/Q_T	E. Hemodynamic monitoring device placed in the pulmonary artery.
	F. Amount of wasted ventilation per breath.
4. _____ Apache score	G. Techniques for lung mapping.
	H. Popular acute illness index.
5. _____ V_D/V_T	I. Bedside test for respiratory muscle strength.
	J. Physiologic shunt.
6. _____ EIT and ARM	
7. _____ Preload	
8. _____ Maximal inspiratory pressure	
9. _____ Glasgow Coma Scale score	
10. _____ Artifacts	

PRINCIPLES OF MONITORING

Monitoring Oxygenation

11. Describe the difference between noninvasive and invasive monitoring.

12. How are exchange of oxygen and the removal of carbon dioxide best monitored invasively? What noninvasive test can be used for immediate continuous assessment of oxygenation?

   A. Invasive: _____

   B. Noninvasive: _____

Copyright © 2025, Elsevier, Inc. All rights reserved.

13. Tissue oxygenation depends on several factors. List four of them.

    A. _____

    B. _____

    C. _____

    D. _____

14. What are the most serious clinical limitations of using pulse oximetry to assess respiratory status?

    _____

15. What is tissue oxygen sensing?

    _____

16. What does the Fick equation measure?

    _____

17. How are the following measurements useful when monitoring an ICU patient?

    A. PaO_2/F_IO_2 ratio: _____

    B. $(P(A - a)O_2)$: _____

    C. OI: _____

18. What does the Berlin Definition of ARDS include?

    A. _____

    B. _____

    C. _____

    D. _____

    E. _____

19. What is the most accurate way to measure oxygenation efficiency? What is the formula?

    A. _____

    B. _____

20. What four factors are included in the Murray lung injury score?

    A. _____

    B. _____

    C. _____

    D. _____

Monitoring Ventilation

21. When is ventilation considered adequate?

    _____

22. Describe a patient in which capnometry would be a useful tool.

Copyright © 2025, Elsevier, Inc. All rights reserved.

23. Measuring physiologic dead space assesses efficiency of ventilation.

State the modified Bohr equation.

$V_D/V_T =$ _____

24. List the normal and critical values for dead space–to–tidal volume ratio.

A. Normal_____   _____

B. Critical is > _____ and predicts failure to wean.

MONITORING LUNG AND CHEST WALL MECHANICS

25. The pressure–volume curve is a ventilator graphic that can show compliance and lower inflection points. The lower inflection point may help you set what ventilator parameter?

_____

26. The upper inflection point may point out what problem?

_____

27. What is normal compliance? How is it calculated?

_____

28. What is the formula for calculating airway resistance?

$R_{aw} =$ _____

29. What is normal airway resistance? What's normal for a ventilated patient?

A. Normal_____

B. Ventilated patients _____

30. What is the safe maximum value for peak pressure? _____

31. What are the maximum safe plateau pressures? _____

32. Explain how adjustment of extrinsic (ventilator) PEEP is related to the level of intrinsic (auto) PEEP.

33. Define stress index. What can it be useful in determining?

34. What is the primary goal of manipulating MAP?

_____

356

Copyright © 2025, Elsevier, Inc. All rights reserved.

Monitoring Breathing Effort and Patterns

35. What is the simplest way to monitor a patient's work of breathing?

_____

36. What is a $P_{0.1}$? What two factors influence this measurement?

_____

37. What are the benefits of measuring MIP compared to VC?

A. _____

B. _____

MONITORING THE PATIENT–VENTILATOR SYSTEM

38. Briefly discuss the areas that are part of a patient-ventilator system check.

A. Airway _____

B. Vent settings _____

C. Gas exchange _____

D. Respiratory mechanics _____

E. The patient _____

F. Alarms _____

G. Other issues _____

39. How can ventilator graphics be used in the patient-ventilator system check?

A. _____

B. _____

C. _____

D. _____

E. _____

40. Explain the key steps listed below regarding a patient-ventilator system check.
A. Before entering the room

B. Explain

Copyright © 2025, Elsevier, Inc. All rights reserved.

C. Observe

D. Drain

E. Airway

F. Inspect

G. Auscultate

H. Note pressures (at least three)

I. Graphics

  Copyright © 2025, Elsevier, Inc. All rights reserved.

41. What is the most common noninvasive tool used to monitor the conduction system of the heart?

42. Identify the two main sites for arterial cannulation in adults.

    A. _____

    B. _____

43. What are the two indications for an indwelling arterial line?

    A. _____

    B. _____

44. List six conditions that suggest insertion of a pulmonary artery catheter.

    A. _____

    B. _____

    C. _____

    D. _____

    E. _____

    F. _____

45. List the normal values for these parameters.

    A. Central venous pressure (CVP) _____

    B. Right atrial pressure (RA) _____

    C. Pulmonary artery_____

        1. Systolic _____

        2. Diastolic_____

    D. Pulmonary artery wedge pressure (PCWP) _____

    E. Cardiac output (CO) _____

    F. Cardiac index (CI) _____

    G. Systemic vascular resistance (SVR) _____

    H. Pulmonary vascular resistance (PVR) _____

46. What common respiratory problem results in vasoconstriction, or elevated vascular resistance in the pulmonary vessels?

    _____

NEUROLOGIC MONITORING

47. Why are the pupils of interest in assessing neurologic status?

    _____

48. Name one of the breathing patterns that suggests a neurologic deficit.

    _____

359

Copyright © 2025, Elsevier, Inc. All rights reserved.

49. Describe what happens to the brain for each of the ICP values below.

    A. 10 to 15 mm Hg _____

    B. 15 to 20 mm Hg _____

    C. 30 to 35 mm Hg _____

50. The Glasgow Coma Scale is a popular tool used to assess acute neurologic deficits. What do the following scores mean?

    A. 9 to 13 _____

    B. <8 _____

MONITORING RENAL AND LIVER FUNCTION

51. Which two tests are commonly used together to monitor renal function?

52. Define polyuria and oliguria in terms of actual daily output.

53. How is liver function usually evaluated?

NUTRITIONAL MONITORING

54. What does the functional nutritional assessment consist of?

55. What is the most frequently used laboratory measure of nutritional status? What value indicates sever malnutrition?

 Copyright © 2025, Elsevier, Inc. All rights reserved.

TROUBLESHOOTING

56. Troubleshooting revolves around which two general problem areas? (See Box 46-12.)

    A. _____

    B. _____

57. Identify common problems and suggest a corrective action.

Clue to Problem	Possible Cause	Corrective Action
Decreased minute ventilation or V_T		
Increased minute ventilation or V_T		
Change in respiratory rate		
Sudden increase in peak airway pressure		
Gradual increase in peak airway pressure		
Sudden decrease in peak airway pressure		
F_iO_2 drift		
Inspired gas temperature too high		
Changes in static pressure		
Changes in ventilator setting		

58. Regardless of the source of the problem, what is always the first priority?

_____

59. If there is any doubt as to the cause or solution of a problem, what action should you take?

WHAT DOES THE NBRC SAY?

Circle the best answer.

60. A 42-year-old patient with a cervical spine injury is being mechanically ventilated in control mode. As you enter the room, the low-pressure alarm is sounding. The patient is connected to the ventilator, but you do not see his chest moving. Your first action would be to _____.
    A. manually ventilate the patient with the resuscitation bag
    B. check the alarm settings
    C. observe the exhaled volumes
    D. manually ventilate the patient with the mechanical ventilator

361

Copyright © 2025, Elsevier, Inc. All rights reserved.

61. After insertion of a Swan-Ganz catheter via the left subclavian vein, a patient's compliance quickly drops. The high-pressure alarm on the ventilator is activated. Breath sounds are absent over the left chest, and the trachea is deviated to the right side. The patient appears extremely anxious. What action should the RCP take?
   A. Use a capnometer to assess ventilation noninvasively.
   B. Recommend administration of Versed.
   C. Call for a portable chest radiograph.
   D. Recommend chest tube insertion.

62. A 38-year-old woman with a diagnosis of myasthenia gravis is being mechanically ventilated. As you enter the room, the high-pressure alarm is sounding. The patient appears anxious. Auscultation reveals coarse bilateral rhonchi. What action should you take at this time?
   A. Manually ventilate the patient.
   B. Check the alarm setting.
   C. Recommend sedation.
   D. Suction the patient.

63. A 77-year-old woman with emphysema is being mechanically ventilated. The high-pressure and high-rate alarms are being activated. Breath sounds are clear. Pulse oximetry and vital sign values are within normal limits. Hemodynamics are normal. ABGs are stable. The patient is very agitated, and her respiratory rate is 32. What are your recommendations?
   A. Administer Versed.
   B. Increase the alarm limit.
   C. Suction the patient.
   D. Call for a portable chest radiograph.

64. The data below are reported for a patient:

   PCWP   25 mm Hg
   PAP   40/24 mm Hg
   CI   1.9 L/min/m^2

   These data suggest which of the following?
   A. Noncardiogenic pulmonary edema
   B. Cardiogenic pulmonary edema
   C. Pulsus paradoxus
   D. Hypovolemia

65. When properly placed, the distal tip of the Swan-Ganz catheter will be located in the _____.
   A. left atrium
   B. right atrium
   C. right ventricle
   D. pulmonary artery

Questions 66 through 68 refer to the following situation:
   A patient is intubated and placed on the ventilator after she develops respiratory failure following hip replacement surgery. The following values are recorded:

   $PaCO_2$ 50 mm Hg
   PaO_2 60 mm Hg
   F_IO_2 0.40
   $PECO_2$ 10 mm Hg
   Tidal volume   800 ml
   Respiratory rate   20

66. These data indicate a dead space to tidal volume ratio of _____.
   A. 20%
   B. 40%
   C. 60%
   D. 80%

  Copyright © 2025, Elsevier, Inc. All rights reserved.

67. What is the exhaled minute volume?
    A. 8.0 L
    B. 12.0 L
    C. 16.0 L
    D. 20.0 L

68. What is the alveolar minute volume?
    A. 3.2 L
    B. 11.2 L
    C. 12.8 L
    D. 16.0 L

69. The following information is recorded for a patient:

    $\dot{V}O_2$ 200 ml/min
    CaO_2 16 vol %
    CvO_2 12 vol %

    What is the cardiac output?
    A. 2.0 L/min
    B. 3.0 L/min
    C. 4.0 L/min
    D. 5.0 L/min

70. The hemodynamic data below are recorded for a patient who is being mechanically ventilated.

    Cardiac output   3.5 L/min
    PAP   16/8 mm Hg
    PCWP   4 mm Hg
    CVP   2 mm Hg
    HR   125/min

    These data probably indicate _____.
    A. hypovolemia
    B. pulmonary hypertension
    C. fluid overload
    D. pulmonary embolism

FOOD FOR THOUGHT

Vascular access and line placement is becoming the responsibility of the respiratory therapist. Do some research. What is the VA-BC credential? In your state, who places invasive lines? Does your area of practice utilize RTs on "line teams?"

Copyright © 2025, Elsevier, Inc. All rights reserved.

53 Discontinuing Ventilatory Support

WORD WIZARD

Please write the meaning of these terms.

ASV _____

ATC _____

MMV _____

PSV _____

PMV _____

RSBI _____

SBT _____

SAT _____

REASONS FOR VENTILATOR DEPENDENCE

1. Define ventilator dependence.

2. What's the difference between weaning from a ventilator and ventilator discontinuation?

    A. Weaning _____

    B. Ventilator discontinuation (liberation) _____

3. List the five general categories that patients who are being considered for removal from ventilatory support fall into.

    A. _____

    B. _____

    C. _____

    D. _____

4. List four factors that determine total ventilatory workload.

    A. _____

    B. _____

    C. _____

    D. _____

Copyright © 2025, Elsevier, Inc. All rights reserved.

5. Give examples of conditions that adversely affect ventilatory capacity.

A. CNS drive

   1. _____

   2. _____

   3. _____

   4. _____

B. Muscle strength

   1. _____

   2. _____

   3. _____

   4. _____

6. Successful discontinuation of ventilatory support is related to which patient's condition?

A. _____

B. _____

C. _____

D. _____

PATIENT EVALUATION

7. What is the first thing you should evaluate whether you are considering weaning or taking the patient off the ventilator? *The single most important thing.*

_____

8. What are the four questions you should ask?

A. _____

B. _____

C. _____

D. _____

365

Copyright © 2025, Elsevier, Inc. All rights reserved.

9. Your board examinations will expect you to identify these classic criteria for weaning from mechanical ventilation. Fill in the criterion values below.

Measurement	Criterion
A. $PaCO_2$	_____
B. pH	_____
C. VC (ml/kg)	_____
D. Spontaneous V_T	_____
E. Spontaneous rate	_____
F. V_E	_____
G. MVV	_____
H. MIF (NIF, MIP)	_____
I. V_D/V_T	_____
J. $P(A - a)O_2$ on 100%	_____
K. P/F ratio	_____
L. PaO_2	_____
M. Qs/Qt	_____
N. F_iO_2	_____
O. f/V_T	_____
P. Compliance	_____

10. Physical assessment of respiratory muscles may be useful. Describe what you are looking for in this area.

11. Rapid shallow breathing index may be the best overall predictor of weaning outcomes. Calculate the rapid shallow breathing index for a patient who has a spontaneous rate of 25 with a spontaneous volume of 350 ml. What are the criteria for success?

    A. Formula _____

    B. Calculation _____

    C. Criteria _____

12. Give the PaO_2, F_iO_2, and PEEP values that should be met prior to weaning.

    A. PaO_2 _____

    B. F_iO_2 _____

    C. PEEP _____

Copyright © 2025, Elsevier, Inc. All rights reserved.

13. Describe the ways that renal function may affect weaning.

A. Electrolytes _____

B. Fluid balance and urine output _____

C. Metabolic acidosis _____

14. Describe the ideal CNS status needed for discontinuation to be successful.

15. Explain the following indices for weaning:

CROP score: _____

Adverse Factor/Ventilator Score: _____

Weaning index: _____

Burns Weaning Assessment Program: _____

16. What turns out to be the best indices?

_____

17. How can the RT improve conditions in the airway?

_____

18. What environmental considerations should be taken?

_____

WEANING METHODS

19. List the three basic methods of discontinuing ventilatory support.

A. _____

B. _____

C. _____

20. Describe the specific advantage of using the ventilator instead of the T-tube.

_____

21. What is the typical minimum length of time for a spontaneous trial when you are going for rapid discontinuance?

_____

22. What does research show about SIMV as it compares to SBTs?

_____

Copyright © 2025, Elsevier, Inc. All rights reserved.

23. From what level of PSV may a patient be extubated?

_____

24. What is an SAT? Why do we do it?

25. When should you repeat the SBT if the patient fails the first trial?

_____

NEWER TECHNIQUES FOR FACILITATING VENTILATOR DISCONTINUANCE

26. Describe mandatory minute ventilation (MMV).

_____

27. Describe adaptive support ventilation (ASV).

28. Why is there a desire to develop a computer-based weaning protocol?

29. When in the weaning process should mobilization of a patient begin?

MONITORING THE PATIENT DURING WEANING

30. What are the two easily monitored and reliable indicators of patient progress during weaning?

    A. _____

    B. _____

31. What is the simplest way to monitor oxygenation during weaning?

Copyright © 2025, Elsevier, Inc. All rights reserved.

32. Give the expected and excessive changes for each of the following parameters.

Parameter	Expected	Deleterious
A. Respiratory rate	_____	_____
B. PaO_2	_____	_____
C. $PaCO_2$	_____	_____
D. Heart rate	_____	_____
E. Blood pressure	_____	_____

EXTUBATION

33. What is the minimum ability required for personnel performing routine extubation?

_____

34. What is the minimum ability required for personnel performing high-risk extubation?

_____

35. What are common patient complaints following extubation?

VENTILATOR DISCONTINUANCE FAILURE

36. Identify five common causes of weaning failure.

A. _____

B. _____

C. _____

D. _____

E. _____

37. What are the alternative care sites for the long-term ventilator patient?

38. Who should be involved in the decision to terminate life support?

39. Discuss the three factors mentioned in your text used to help make the decision.

Copyright © 2025, Elsevier, Inc. All rights reserved.

A 61-year-old woman is placed on the ventilator for respiratory failure for CHF and COPD. Twenty-four hours later, the physician asks for your recommendation regarding weaning. Breath sounds reveal coarse crackles in both bases. Pedal edema is present as well. The following information is obtained.

Spontaneous RR	28
Spontaneous V_T	0.2 L
MIF	−18 cm H_2O
VC	0.6 L
HR	116
BP	90/60
pH	7.33
$PaCO_2$	35 mm Hg
PaO_2	65 (on F_iO_2 0.5)
Cardiac index	2.3

40. What is your assessment of her respiratory status?

41. Has the primary problem been resolved?

42. What is the rapid shallow breathing index?

43. Explain your recommendation regarding initiating weaning. If you recommend weaning, also recommend the method.

Copyright © 2025, Elsevier, Inc. All rights reserved.

A 61-year-old man is placed on the ventilator following open-heart surgery. Twelve hours later, the patient is awake, and the physician asks for your recommendation regarding weaning. The following information is obtained:

Spontaneous RR	14
Spontaneous V_T	0.2 L
MIF	−35 cm H_2O
VC	1.2 L
HR	116
BP	90/60
pH	7.37
$PaCO_2$	35 mm Hg
PaO_2	85 (on F_iO_2 0.35)

44. What is your assessment of his respiratory status?

45. Has the primary problem been resolved?

46. What is the rapid shallow breathing index?

47. Explain your recommendation regarding initiating weaning. If you recommend weaning, also recommend a technique.

Copyright © 2025, Elsevier, Inc. All rights reserved.

A 61-year-old is placed on the ventilator following an acute episode of Guillain-Barré syndrome. Twenty-one days later, the patient is regaining strength and movement in his limbs. The physician asks for your recommendation regarding weaning. The following information is obtained:

Spontaneous RR	22
Spontaneous V_T	0.22 L
MIF	−20 cm H_2O
VC	1.0 L
HR	116
BP	90/60
pH	7.38
$PaCO_2$	37 mm Hg
PaO_2	70 (on F_iO_2 0.40)

48. What is your assessment of his respiratory status?

49. Has the primary problem been resolved?

50. What is the rapid shallow breathing index?

51. Explain your recommendation regarding initiating weaning. If you recommend weaning, also recommend a technique.

A 5-foot 2-inch, 50-kg, 80-year-old woman has been on the ventilator for 2 days because of hemodynamic instability following open-heart surgery. The vitals are now stable. The physician wants you to conduct a spontaneous breathing trial. You suction the patient and sit her up for trial. Pretrial respiratory rate is 22, MIP is −45 mm Hg, and spontaneous volume is 400 ml. She is placed on a T-piece for 3 minutes with 40% oxygen. After 3 minutes, the f is 25, MIP is −40, and V_T is 420.

52. What would you recommend at this time?

53. What is the RSBI?

54. How long does she need to succeed on the trial before you would consider extubation?

Copyright © 2025, Elsevier, Inc. All rights reserved.

Circle the best answer.

55. Which of the following would you evaluate prior to initiating weaning?
    1. PaO$_2$
    2. Gag reflex
    3. Spontaneous respiratory rate
    4. Urine output

    A. 1 and 2 only
    B. 1 and 3 only
    C. 2 and 4 only
    D. 3 and 4 only

56. A patient being assessed for readiness for weaning has the following values:

pH	7.36
PaCO$_2$	42 mm Hg
PaO$_2$	67 mm Hg (F$_i$O$_2$ 40%)
MIP	−25 cm H$_2$O
Pulse	105
Respirations	20
VC	12 ml/kg

    What action should the RT recommend at this time?
    A. Initiate a CPAP trial.
    B. Continue with mechanical ventilation.
    C. Initiate breathing exercises to strengthen ventilatory muscles.
    D. Repeat the vital capacity maneuver.

57. Which of the following indicates a readiness to wean?
    A. Spontaneous rate of 28
    B. Spontaneous tidal volume of 200 ml
    C. Negative inspiratory force of 18 cm H$_2$O
    D. Minute volume of 8 L/min

58. An alert patient is being mechanically ventilated. Settings are:

Mode	SIMV
Rate	2
Tidal volume (set)	500
F$_i$O$_2$	0.30
PEEP	5 cm H$_2$O

    ABG results 30 minutes after initiating these settings are:

pH	7.37
PaCO$_2$	38 mm Hg
PaO$_2$	75 mm Hg

    What should the RT recommend at this time?
    A. Increase the set rate to 4.
    B. Discontinue mechanical ventilation.
    C. Decrease the PEEP to 2 cm H$_2$O.
    D. Decrease the F$_i$O$_2$ to 0.21.

Copyright © 2025, Elsevier, Inc. All rights reserved.

59. A patient is being ventilated in the SIMV mode with a rate of 8, volume of 800, and F_iO_2 of 0.40. ABG results show:

pH 7.47
$PaCO_2$ 33 mm Hg
PaO_2 88 mm Hg
HCO_3^- 23 mEq/L

What action should the RT recommend in response to these findings?
A. Increase the tidal volume.
B. Increase the F_iO_2.
C. Change to AC mode.
D. Reduce the rate.

60. A patient on SIMV experiences difficulty each time you try to reduce the rate below 6. The patient becomes tachypneic with a rate of 28 and a spontaneous volume of 200. Which of the following modifications would be *least* useful in this situation?
A. Adding pressure support ventilation
B. Transfer back to full ventilatory support
C. Extubation
D. Change to flow triggering

FOOD FOR THOUGHT

61. What is the single best approach to weaning?

Copyright © 2025, Elsevier, Inc. All rights reserved.

54 Neonatal and Pediatric Respiratory Care

WORD WIZARD

WORD WIZARD

Write out the words to these acronyms.

AGA _____

CPAP _____

ECMO _____

HFV _____

INO _____

PPHN _____

PDA _____

ROP _____

FETAL ASSESSMENT

1. Assessment of the newborn begins with maternal history. Identify three conditions that are likely to result in a baby who is small for its gestational age.

    A. _____

    B. _____

    C. _____

2. Identify five maternal factors likely to lead to premature delivery.

    A. _____

    B. _____

    C. _____

    D. _____

    E. _____

3. What maternal metabolic condition is likely to result in an infant who is large for its gestational age?

    _____

Copyright © 2025, Elsevier, Inc. All rights reserved.

4. Briefly describe each of the following tests.
   A. Ultrasonography

   B. Amniocentesis

   C. Fetal heart rate monitoring (Be sure to discuss accelerations, decelerations, and heart rate values and what they mean.)

   D. Fetal scalp blood gas analysis (Include normal values and describe the relationship between fetal scalp gases and arterial blood gases.)

NEWBORN ASSESSMENT

5. When are Apgar scores taken? _____

6. Fill in the chart regarding the Apgar scoring system.

	SIGN	0	1	2
A.	Heart rate			
B.	Respiration			
C.	Muscle tone			
D.	Reflex			
E.	Color			

Copyright © 2025, Elsevier, Inc. All rights reserved.

7. What term is used to describe the following weeks of gestation?

   A. Before 38 weeks _____

   B. 38 to 42 weeks _____

   C. After 42 weeks _____

8. Name the two common systems used for assessing gestational age based on physical characteristics and neurologic signs.

   A. _____

   B. _____

9. Explain the abbreviations and identify the weights that correspond to the following terms.

	ABBREVIATION	FULL NAME	WEIGHTS/PERCENTS
A.	VLBW		
B.	LBW		
C.	AGA		
D.	LGA		
E.	SGA		

ASSESSING THE NEWBORN

10. State the normal range for a full-term infant's vital signs.

    A. Heart rate _____

    B. Respiratory rate _____

    C. Blood pressure _____

11. Explain the significance of each sign.

    A. Nasal flaring _____

    B. Cyanosis _____

    C. Expiratory grunting _____

    D. Retractions _____

    E. Paradoxical breathing _____

12. What scoring system is used to grade the severity of underlying lung disease?

    _____

13. How is the need for surfactant determined?

Copyright © 2025, Elsevier, Inc. All rights reserved.

14. What are the two usual sites for obtaining blood gas samples in infants?

A. _____

B. _____

15. List the ABG values for preterm and term infants at birth.

	PARAMETER	PRETERM (1 TO 5 HOURS)	NORMAL TERM (5 HOURS)	NORMAL PRETERM INFANTS (5 DAYS)
A.	pH			
B.	$PaCO_2$			
C.	PaO_2			

RESPIRATORY CARE TECHNIQUES

16. Considering its hazards, we need to agree on the safe limits for oxygen therapy. Give the accepted ranges for these parameters.

A. F_1O_2 < _____ %

B. Preemie SpO_2 _____ to _____

17. How could oxygen cause heart problems to worsen in some newborns?

18. Compare the use of the following oxygen delivery devices.

	DEVICE	AGE	ADVANTAGE	DISADVANTAGE
A.	AEM			
B.	Cannula			
C.	Incubator			
D.	Hood			
E.	Tent			

19. Name four conditions in which secretion retention is common in children.

A. _____

B. _____

C. _____

D. _____

Copyright © 2025, Elsevier, Inc. All rights reserved.

20. Why is it so important to monitor ALL aspects of infants who need bronchial hygiene therapy?

21. What type of device is used for patients who are intubated?

_____

22. In terms of humidification, what's important about volume and water level for babies on ventilators?

23. What factors could affect the delivery of humidity from a servo-controlled heated humidifier to an infant who is mechanically ventilated?

24. State the four methods you can use to deliver aerosol medications to children.

A. _____

B. _____

C. _____

D. _____

AIRWAY MANAGEMENT

25. Identify the correct ET size and suction catheter size for these children.

	AGE/WEIGHT	ET INTERNAL DIAMETER (ID)	LENGTH (ORAL)	SUCTION
A.	<1000 g			
B.	1000 to 2000 g			
C.	2000 to 3000 g			
D.	>3000 g			
E.	2 years			
F.	6 years			

Copyright © 2025, Elsevier, Inc. All rights reserved.

26. State the two formulas for calculating tube diameter.

27. What is the consequence of placing an ET tube that is too small in an infant?

28. Estimate the correct tube size for a 4-year-old using the first formula in question 26.

29. Which laryngoscope blade is usually used for infant intubation?

   _____

30. Which airway can be used as an alternative to intubation in children?

31. What are the recommended vacuum pressures for suctioning infants and children?

   A. Infants _____

   B. Children _____

32. Identify the criteria for initiating chest compressions after delivery.

   _____

CONTINUOUS POSITIVE AIRWAY PRESSURE

33. What is the specific indication for CPAP? Give the blood gas values.

   A. Indication _____

   B. Blood gas values _____

Copyright © 2025, Elsevier, Inc. All rights reserved.

34. Discuss adjustment of CPAP in infants.
    A. Start at

    B. Adjust in increments of

HIGH-FLOW NASAL CANNULA

35. What is the range of flow given for the new cannulas?

   _____

36. What problem may occur if the prongs on a high-flow system fit tightly in the nares?

MECHANICAL VENTILATION

37. What pulmonary diseases typically require mechanical ventilation?

    A. _____

    B. _____

    C. _____

    D. _____

38. Give the range of PIP for infants for initiating time-cycled, pressure-limited ventilation.

   _____

39. Identify the inspiratory time ranges that should be set for these age groups.

    A. Neonates_____

    B. Older children _____

40. What PEEP levels are usually used in neonates for initiating ventilation?

   _____

41. What range of volumes is normally used when volume ventilation is selected?

   _____

Copyright © 2025, Elsevier, Inc. All rights reserved.

42. Why would it be common to observe lower exhaled than inhaled volumes in pediatric patients?

_____

43. List five considerations made prior to extubation.

A. _____

B. _____

C. _____

D. _____

E. _____

HIGH-FREQUENCY VENTILATION

44. Identify the two common characteristics of HFV.

A. V_T _____

B. Rate _____

45. What are the three types of HFV? Which is more common?

A. _____

B. _____

C. _____

Most common? _____

46. How would you wean a patient from HFV?

SPECIALTY GASES

47. What effect does INO have on oxygenation?

_____

48. Two big problems exist with NO inhalation. Explain.
    A. Rebound pulmonary hypertension

    B. Altered hemoglobin

Copyright © 2025, Elsevier, Inc. All rights reserved.

49. Why is heliox typically used? When is it less effective?

WHAT DOES THE NBRC SAY?

Circle the best answer.

50. Which of the following tests would be useful in determining lung maturity?
    A. Sweat chloride
    B. Phosphatidylglycerol levels
    C. Fetal hemoglobin
    D. Pneumogram

51. Calculate the Apgar score for a crying infant who has a heart rate of 120, actively moves, and sneezes when a catheter is put in the nose but has blue extremities.
    A. 5
    B. 6
    C. 7
    D. 9

52. The simplest way to apply CPAP to treat hypoxemia in an infant is to use _____.
    A. nasal prongs
    B. nasal mask
    C. full-face mask
    D. oxygen hood

53. Excessive oxygen delivery to newborns may raise the risk of
    A. pneumonia.
    B. retinopathy of prematurity.
    C. cystic fibrosis.
    D. PPHN.

54. What vacuum pressure would you set for suctioning a newborn?
    A. Suction pressure should not exceed 80 mm Hg.
    B. Suction pressure should not exceed 100 mmHg.
    C. Suction pressure should not exceed 120 mmHg.
    D. Newborns should not be suctioned.

55. What size endotracheal tube would you recommend for a 1500-g preemie?
    A. 2.5
    B. 3.0
    C. 3.5
    D. 4.0

FOOD FOR THOUGHT

If you choose to work in this field, it would be a good idea to take the Neonatal/Pediatric Specialist Examination to test your knowledge and demonstrate your competence in this specialty area.

Copyright © 2025, Elsevier, Inc. All rights reserved.

55 Patient Education and Health Promotion

WORD WIZARD

Write out the definition for each of these terms.

1. Affective domain _____

2. Cognitive domain _____

3. Health education _____

4. Health promotion _____

5. Psychomotor domain _____

PATIENT EDUCATION

6. List the top four causes of death in the United States.

   1. _____

   2. _____

   3. _____

   4. _____

7. Why is educating the public about these illnesses so important?

   _____

8. Why should the development of written objectives for patient teaching be considered?

   _____

9. How can the RT state an objective in measurable terms during patient education sessions?

   A. Begin with a _____

   B. Write an action _____

   C. Add a condition _____

   D. Write a standard _____

10. Give an example of an objective for each of the following learning domains.

	DOMAIN	OBJECTIVE
A.	Cognitive	
B.	Affective	
C.	Psychomotor	

385

Copyright © 2025, Elsevier, Inc. All rights reserved.

11. Which of the learning domains should be evaluated before you proceed with patient education?

_____

12. What is the key to motivating patients to learn?

_____

13. What is the key to teaching psychomotor skills? How can you confirm that a patient or family member has learned a new skill?

_____

14. Give an example from the text of how to relate psychomotor skills a patient uses every day to help make the transition from everyday life to therapy.

_____

Teaching Children, Adolescents, Adults, and Older Adults

15. How is teaching a child different from teaching an adult? How is it the same?

16. Where could you find resource materials to help in teaching children with asthma?

_____

17. What suggestions are given for rewarding performance?

Evaluation

18. What process answers the question "Has the patient learned?" When should you begin to develop this process?

19. Describe some of the formal and informal ways you can tell if a patient has met affective domain objectives.

Copyright © 2025, Elsevier, Inc. All rights reserved.

20. What is the primary goal of health education?

21. Learning activities must incorporate values and beliefs of the learner. List four factors that need to be considered in this area.

    A. _____

    B. _____

    C. _____

    D. _____

22. How do the personal characteristics of the educator impact learning?

HEALTH PROMOTION AND CHRONIC DISEASE MANAGEMENT

23. Compare the standard medical approach to health in the United States with the public health model.

24. What are the broad goals of the Healthy People 2030 initiative?

25. Discuss how RTs might participate in the management of COPD through education.

Copyright © 2025, Elsevier, Inc. All rights reserved.

26. Besides the hospital, name four other settings where RTs would be likely to function as individual counselors or public health advocates.

A. _____

B. _____

C. _____

D. _____

CASE STUDIES

Your text has several good cases in the form of "Mini-Clinis," so let's do something else. Suppose you had to teach your classmates how to use a peak flow meter. Write three objectives for this topic for each domain using behavioral terms.

27. Cognitive domain

A.

B.

C.

28. Affective domain

A.

B.

C.

Copyright © 2025, Elsevier, Inc. All rights reserved.

29. Psychomotor domain

    A.

    B.

    C.

30. How long would your teaching session last?

    _____

31. Give examples of how you would involve the following in your session.

    A. Hearing _____

    B. Seeing _____

    C. Touching _____

    D. Writing _____

    E. Speaking _____

32. Give an example of how you would measure learning for each domain.

    A. Cognitive _____

    B. Affective _____

    C. Psychomotor _____

WHAT DOES THE NBRC SAY?

33. The best way to ensure that a patient has learned to properly administer a bronchodilator via MDI is to
    A. ask the patient to answer questions regarding inhaler use.
    B. give the patient appropriate literature regarding MDI use.
    C. ask the patient to demonstrate how to use the inhaler.
    D. have the patient explain when he is to use the MDI.

Copyright © 2025, Elsevier, Inc. All rights reserved.

34. Which of the following best describes the application of the best health care practices to a population diagnosed with a chronic illness one person at a time?
    A. Disease management
    B. Population health
    C. Health literacy
    D. Chronic care

FOOD FOR THOUGHT

35. Why do you think the public should be educated about the risk factors for the top causes of death?

36. Describe the patient-centered care approach.

Copyright © 2025, Elsevier, Inc. All rights reserved.

56 Cardiopulmonary Rehabilitation

Match the following terms and acronyms to their definitions.

Terms and Acronyms	Definitions
1. _____ ADL	A. Physical activities designed to strengthen muscles and improve O_2 utilization.
2. _____ Borg scale	B. Measure of an individual's ability to perform common tasks.
3. _____ CORF	C. Point where there is insufficient O_2 to meet the demands of energy metabolism.
4. _____ Karvonen's formula	D. Measure of an individual's perception of breathing difficulty.
5. _____ Progressive resistance	E. Cardiac goal for aerobic conditioning based on 65% of maximum O_2 consumption.
6. _____ OBLA	F. Ratio of CO_2 production to O_2 consumption.
7. _____ Reconditioning	G. Medicare-approved facility that provides ambulatory rehabilitation services.
8. _____ Respiratory quotient	H. Common method used to calculate target heart rate for exercise.
9. _____ Target heart rate	I. Training method that gradually increases muscle workloads.

DEFINITIONS AND GOALS

10. What event placed a focus on hospital readmissions and the importance of pulmonary rehabilitation?

11. In your own words, define pulmonary rehabilitation.

12. List three general goals of pulmonary rehabilitation?

A. _____

B. _____

C. _____

Copyright © 2025, Elsevier, Inc. All rights reserved.

13. How do clinical and social sciences play a role in establishing ways to improve the patient's quality of life?

14. Define OBLA and describe it relation to physical reconditioning.

15. How can you estimate MVV using simple spirometry?

_____

16. Identify the three general ways that reconditioning will increase exercise tolerance.

A. _____

B. _____

C. _____

17. Compare the roles of psychosocial and physical methods in terms of outcomes of rehabilitation.

18. Describe the two-way relationship of physical reconditioning and psychosocial support.

STRUCTURE OF A PULMONARY REHABILITATION PROGRAM

19. Why is it so important to have specific objectives for the program goals? How should these objectives be stated?

A.

B.

Copyright © 2025, Elsevier, Inc. All rights reserved.

20. List five accepted benefits of exercise reconditioning.

A. _____

B. _____

C. _____

D. _____

E. _____

21. Research literature clearly shows that rehabilitation has proven benefits. What is the effect of rehabilitation on the progression of the disease?

22. Name three common goals (*not objectives*) for rehabilitation programs.

A. _____

B. _____

C. _____

23. Who manages the overall care in a program and screens the prospective patients?

_____

24. What is the first step in patient evaluation for a pulmonary rehab program?

_____

25. List four tests that should be included with the physical examination.

A. _____

B. _____

C. _____

D. _____

26. Two tests are usually conducted to assess cardiopulmonary status. State two purposes for these tests.

A. Exercise evaluation

1. _____

2. _____

B. Pulmonary function testing

1. _____

2. _____

27. List two contraindications to exercise testing.

_____

_____

393

Copyright © 2025, Elsevier, Inc. All rights reserved.

28. Identify four physiologic parameters that should be monitored during exercise testing.

A. _____

B. _____

C. _____

D. _____

29. List four general groups of patients included in pulmonary rehabilitation programs.

A. _____

B. _____

C. _____

D. _____

30. What are the benefits of grouping patients together on the basis of severity and overall ability?

31. Give one benefit and one drawback of the open-ended program model.

A. Benefit: _____

B. Drawback: _____

32. Give one benefit and one drawback to the traditional closed design.

A. Benefit: _____

B. Drawback: _____

33. Describe Medicare coverage for pulmonary rehabilitation.

34. Describe two ways to set target heart rate for patient exercise.

A. Formula _____

B. Estimate _____

35. Describe a typical walking exercise program. What is our minimum walk time?

 Copyright © 2025, Elsevier, Inc. All rights reserved.

36. What is the basic concept behind ventilatory muscle training?

37. Briefly discuss the following high-priority program educational components.

    A. Breathing control

    B. Stress management

    C. Medications

    D. Diet

38. What is the ideal class size for a rehabilitation program? What external factor affects this ideal?

Copyright © 2025, Elsevier, Inc. All rights reserved.

39. Give specific examples for each of the following sources of program reimbursement.

A. Nongovernment health insurance _____

B. Federal and state health insurance _____

C. Ancillary insurance _____

D. Other options _____

40. What is/are the most likely cause(s) of lack of measurable improvement within a pulmonary rehabilitation program?

41. Potential hazards do exist in pulmonary rehabilitation. Give one from each category:

A. Cardio _____

B. Blood gas _____

C. Muscular _____

D. Miscellaneous _____

CASE STUDIES

Case 1

An alert 55-year-old man with long-standing asthma and COPD is admitted for acute exacerbation of his illness following a "chest cold." This is the fourth admission for this patient in the past 3 months. He tells you that he has had to quit his job and take early retirement because of his lung problems.

42. What concerns does this situation raise?

43. Explain the benefits of entering a rehabilitation program to this patient.

Copyright © 2025, Elsevier, Inc. All rights reserved.

A 57-year-old woman with chronic bronchitis is enrolled in your pulmonary rehabilitation program. During walking exercises, she complains of dyspnea and will not continue with the walk.

44. What assessments would be useful in this situation?

45. Give several possible methods for modifying the exercise program to improve this patient's compliance.

WHAT DOES THE NBRC SAY?

Circle the answers.

46. A COPD patient has enrolled in a pulmonary rehabilitation program. The patient should be informed that the program will help provide all of the benefits *except* _____.
    A. increased physical endurance
    B. improved PFT results
    C. increased activity levels
    D. improved cardiovascular function

47. During an exercise test a patient is able to reach a maximum heart rate of 120. His resting heart rate is 70. What target heart rate would you recommend for this patient during aerobic conditioning?
    A. 70 beats per minute
    B. 85 beats per minute
    C. 100 beats per minute
    D. 115 beats per minute

48. Which of the following tests would be useful in assessing ventilatory reserve during exercise testing?
    A. Forced vital capacity
    B. Maximum voluntary ventilation
    C. Body plethysmography
    D. Single breath nitrogen washout

Copyright © 2025, Elsevier, Inc. All rights reserved.

All throughout *Egan's* we find references to the Borg scale. This scale is a valuable tool that can be easily used at the bedside or in the rehabilitation setting.

49. Describe the Borg scale. What is the value of this instrument?

50. Compare and contrast cardiac rehabilitation with pulmonary rehabilitation.

Copyright © 2025, Elsevier, Inc. All rights reserved.

57 Respiratory Care in Alternative Settings

WORD WIZARD

Write out the meanings of the following acronyms.

1. CMS _____

2. DMEPOS _____

3. NIV _____

4. LTACH _____

5. SNF _____

6. TTOT _____

MORE RECENT DEVELOPMENTS AND TRENDS

7. What is the most common alternative site for health care?

   _____

8. How has the Patient Protection and Affordable Care Act (ACA) of 2010 affected alternative settings?

RELEVANT TERMS AND GOALS

9. List five areas of nonacute or alternative care.

   A. _____

   B. _____

   C. _____

   D. _____

   E. _____

10. Describe the LTACH and its relationship to respiratory care.

Copyright © 2025, Elsevier, Inc. All rights reserved.

11. What is subacute care?

12. List four common respiratory care services provided in alternative settings.

   A. _____

   B. _____

   C. _____

   D. _____

13. List three of the benefits of respiratory home care.

   A. _____

   B. _____

   C. _____

   Now list three typical disease states that need our help.

   D. _____

   E. _____

   F. _____

STANDARDS

14. What is the purpose of the Medicare Provider Certification Program?

15. Who is responsible for accreditation of companies that provide home care services?

   _____

16. What do RTs like about working in alternative care settings?

400

Copyright © 2025, Elsevier, Inc. All rights reserved.

17. Compare traditional and alternative settings in terms of the following areas.

AREA	TRADITIONAL	ALTERNATIVE
A. Diagnostic tests		
B. Equipment		
C. Supervision		
D. Patient assessment		
E. Work schedule		
F. Time constraints		

DISCHARGE PLANNING

18. Explain the role of the following practitioners in the alternative care setting team.

A. Utilization and review _____

B. Social services _____

C. Physical therapy _____

D. Psychiatrist _____

E. DME supplier _____

19. How can you confirm that a nonprofessional caregiver is able to perform care?

_____

20. Discuss items in the home environment that must be assessed prior to discharge.

A. Accessibility

B. Equipment

C. Environment

OXYGEN THERAPY

21. Why do so many people use oxygen in alternative care settings in the United States?

_____

401

Copyright © 2025, Elsevier, Inc. All rights reserved.

22. State two of the documented benefits of long-term oxygen therapy.

    A. _____

    B. _____

23. Describe the six elements that must be included in a home oxygen prescription.

    A. _____

    B. _____

    C. _____

    D. _____

    E. _____

    F. _____

24. The AARC Clinical Practice Guidelines for Oxygen in the Home clearly states the indications for oxygen outside the acute care hospital.

    A. Adults, etc., >28 days PaO_2 ≤ _____ mm Hg, or SaO_2 ≤ _____.

    B. Cor pulmonale, CHF, or critical >56% PaO_2 ≤ _____ or SaO_2 ≤ _____.

    C. Ambulation, sleep, or exercise if SaO_2 falls below _____%.

25. What are the two primary uses of compressed oxygen cylinders in alternative settings?

    A. E cylinder _____

    B. H cylinder (or M) _____

26. How do flowmeters used in alternative settings differ from those used in the hospital?

    _____

27. What is the typical range of oxygen percentage a concentrator will supply?

    A. 1 to 2 L/min _____

    B. >5 L/min _____

28. What effect will the concentrator have on a patient's electrical bill?

    _____

29. Describe some of the methods for avoiding communication problems with patients receiving home oxygen therapy.

    _____

30. List at least four areas that should be evaluated when checking a home patient's oxygen concentrator.

    A. _____

    B. _____

    C. _____

    D. _____

Copyright © 2025, Elsevier, Inc. All rights reserved.

31. When a patient is placed on an oxygen-conserving device, how would you determine the correct liter flow to use?

32. What actions should a patient who is wearing transtracheal oxygen take if he believes the catheter isn't working properly?

33. State the three main problems associated with insertion of the transtracheal catheter (see Box 51-4).

A. _____

B. _____

C. _____

34. Describe the basic methods for avoiding complications of transtracheal catheters.

VENTILATORY SUPPORT IN ALTERNATIVE SETTINGS

35. Give examples for each of the three main groups of patients who are placed on ventilators in the alternative care setting.

A. Nocturnal ventilation

1. _____

2. _____

3. _____

B. Continuous mechanical ventilation

1. _____

2. _____

3. _____

C. Terminally ill

1. _____

2. _____

Copyright © 2025, Elsevier, Inc. All rights reserved.

36. Invasive long-term ventilation is always provided via what type of airway?

_____

37. Describe the emergency situations a family must be able to deal with in caring for a home ventilator patient.

38. What options exist for patients who do not want invasive ventilation and cannot use NIV?

39. What options are available on invasive positive pressure ventilator systems during power failures or if a patient wishes to be mobile?

_____

40. What is the biggest challenge associated with NIV?

_____

OTHER MODES OF POSTACUTE VENTILATION IN ALTERNATIVE SITES

41. What is the primary use of bland aerosols in the alternative care setting?

42. What is the major problem with delivery of bland aerosols?

_____

43. What is the most common clinical problem with the CPAP apparatus?

_____

44. Discuss solutions to the common complaint of nasal dryness.

404

   Copyright © 2025, Elsevier, Inc. All rights reserved.

45. Apnea monitors alert parents or caregivers of what three serious signs? How long do they need the monitor?

   A. Condition _____

   B. Duration of monitoring _____

PATIENT ASSESSMENT AND DOCUMENTATION

46. Describe the main areas you would check during initial screening of a patient following admission to an alternative care facility.

47. What areas would be important to assess besides the usual vital signs and evaluation of the respiratory system?

48. How often should a member of the home care team perform a follow-up evaluation for patients receiving respiratory care treatments? What factors should be considered in determining the frequency of visits?

EQUIPMENT DISINFECTION AND MAINTENANCE

49. Describe the process for cleaning a home nebulizer (for example):

   A. _____

   B. _____

   C. _____

50. Describe the guidelines for using water in humidifiers and nebulizers.

Copyright © 2025, Elsevier, Inc. All rights reserved.

51. What is the most important principle of infection control in the home setting?

CASE STUDIES

Case 1

A 70-year-old with COPD is discharged with an order for home oxygen. The room air blood gas prior to discharge is:

pH	7.47
$PaCO_2$	33 mm Hg
PaO_2	62 mm Hg
SaO_2	92%

Medicare returns the CMN as "disapproved" on the basis that this patient does not meet the PO_2 saturation criteria for home oxygen.

52. Make an argument for keeping the patient on oxygen based on your knowledge of respiratory physiology. You won't find a clear answer in the text.

Case 2

A home care patient whom you are seeing uses an oxygen concentrator. He calls you to say that he doesn't think he is getting an adequate amount of flow from his cannula.

53. What are some possible causes of this problem?

54. What would you suggest the patient do to quickly check the cannula?

Copyright © 2025, Elsevier, Inc. All rights reserved.

Case 3

An active 49-year-old with α_1-antitrypsin deficiency is to be discharged with home oxygen. The prescription is for 2 L/min continuous oxygen.

55. What system would you recommend for this patient to use at home?

56. What about a portable system?

WHAT DOES THE NBRC SAY?

Circle the answer.

57. A patient with a tracheostomy is to receive humidification via a nebulizer in his home. With regard to water for the nebulizer, which of the following would be the most appropriate choice for the home setting?
    1. Sterile distilled water should be obtained from the DME provider.
    2. Tap water is sufficient for the home setting if the nebulizer is cleaned properly.
    3. Bottled water can be used as long as it is distilled.
    4. Tap water that is boiled may be used for up to 24 hours.
       A. 1 and 3
       B. 1 and 4
       C. 2 and 3
       D. 2 and 4

58. Which of the following actions would an RT perform during the monthly check of a home oxygen concentrator system?
    1. Replacement of the silica pellets in the sieve bed
    2. Analysis of the F_iO_2 delivered by the concentrator
    3. Filter replacement
    4. Evaluation of the concentrator's electrical system
       A. 1 and 2
       B. 2 and 3
       C. 1 and 4
       D. 3 and 4

59. A patient who is using oxygen at home occasionally needs to go out for health care appointments. What type of portable system would you recommend for this patient?
    A. E cylinder with standard flowmeter.
    B. E cylinder with conserving device.
    C. Small liquid oxygen reservoir.
    D. Patients can go out for short periods without supplemental oxygen.

Copyright © 2025, Elsevier, Inc. All rights reserved.

60. A respiratory care practitioner determines that a cuirass-type negative pressure ventilator is now reading a pressure of −20 cm H_2O when it should be cycling at −35 cm H_2O. The patient is in no distress, but the measured tidal volume

   is 200 ml lower than the desired volume. The practitioner should _____.
   A. begin manual ventilation of the patient
   B. check for leaks in the system
   C. increase the vacuum setting
   D. increase the amount of air in the cuff

FOOD FOR THOUGHT

Think about the care you would want for your mother, father, or even yourself. Wouldn't it be wonderful to be able to care for your loved one (or yourself) safely in a serene environment of an alternative care setting versus a loud, busy hospital?

Copyright © 2025, Elsevier, Inc. All rights reserved.

58 Ethics and End of Life

WORD WIZARD

Write out the meanings of the following acronyms.

1. LST: _____

2. CVVH: _____

3. ECMO: _____

4. SOB: _____

5. PSDA: _____

6. HCA: _____

7. PAS: _____

8. ASBH: _____

9. CIED: _____

10. AICD: _____

11. MCS: _____

12. DNR: _____

13. DNI: _____

MEET THE OBJECTIVES

14. List the three components make up a Goals of Care framework.

   A. _____

   B. _____

   C. _____

15. Define the term 'medical prognosis'.

Copyright © 2025, Elsevier, Inc. All rights reserved.

16. List the questions seeking responses either directly from the patient or from their surrogate decision maker when building the values, beliefs, and preferences component of the Goals of Care framework.

A. _____

B. _____

C. _____

D. _____

E. _____

F. _____

17. What is the purpose of the Patient Self Determination Act (PSDA) Omnibus Reconciliation Act?

18. What happens when a patient has an advance directive and is unable to speak on his/her own behalf?

19. Describe the Doctrine of Double Effect.

20. When terminally extubating a patient, should you provide oxygen? Explain your answer.

FOOD FOR THOUGHT

It is critical for the RT to know what is ethically and legally permissible in the United States and their state of practice related to end-of-life care. Does your hospital offer any training regarding the topic of decision making around life-sustaining treatments and respiratory therapies for critically ill patients? Remember, respiratory therapists should not make assumptions about a patient's or family's wish or preferences and how their unique cultural backgrounds may shape how they arrive at certain decisions.

Copyright © 2025, Elsevier, Inc. All rights reserved.